ACADEMY
FORUM
Third of a Series

EXPERIMENTS AND RESEARCH WITH HUMANS: VALUES IN CONFLICT

NATIONAL ACADEMY OF SCIENCES

WASHINGTON, D.C.   1975

The work upon which this publication is based was performed pursuant to
Contract N01-OD-5-2116, jointly sponsored by the Department of Health,
Education, and Welfare, the National Endowment for the Humanities, and
the National Science Foundation.

International Standard Book Number: 0-309-02347-5

Library of Congress Catalog Card Number: 75-13985

Available from:

Printing and Publishing Office
National Academy of Sciences
2101 Constitution Avenue, N.W.
Washington, D.C.   20418

Printed in the United States of America

FOREWORD

The Forum of the National Academy of Sciences is a public platform for
the appraisal and illumination of broad concerns involving controversy
surrounding the uses of science and technology. This is the record of
the Academy Forum convened on February 18-19, 1975, to consider "Experiments and Research with Humans: Values in Conflict."

In bringing scientists and nonscientists together at one time and in
one place, the Academy Forum projects the proposition that effectively
designed policy and its implementation must recognize the interests and
needs of all relevant constituencies -- private citizens, government,
industry, public interest groups, the scientific community -- the full
spectrum of all those who are responsible for initiating change through
science and those who are affected by it.

A Forum actually begins when a topic is selected. Following the
choice of this particularly complex one by the General Advisory Committee in April of 1974, Dr. Frederick C. Robbins and Dr. Lewis Thomas
agreed to serve as co-chairmen. During the summer the Program Committee, drawn from a wide range of experience and interest, met to define
issues and questions posed by the topic. Throughout the fall and
winter, numerous discussions were held with individuals and groups to
choose speakers and panel participants who would give the broadest
possible frame of reference. Those individuals were then brought together for further discussion. Meanwhile, invitations to attend the
Forum were extended by mail and in the public press to expand the
audience to include the widest possible representation.

This publication presents the culmination of those months of planning when approximately one thousand people came together over the
two-day period in the auditorium of the National Academy of Sciences.
Opinions concerning the success of this Forum undoubtedly are as varied

iii

and as numerous as those who attended it and draw in large part from what was expected of it. Each of the co-chairmen has introduced into the record a retrospective overview of the day he chaired.

In many ways the reader of this volume has an advantage over the participants of the planning and plenary sessions. He is not called upon to make a public statement or compelled to defend a point of view. Removed from the scene of those frequently turbulent two days, he can locate, review, and reformulate the issues; he can observe the wide spectrum of perceptions focused on the subject, identify their sources, and weigh their implications. This opportunity for the reader is basic to our decision to publish an edited proceedings rather than a summary report, which inevitably emerges as only one more view of what took place.

Here, then, in microcosm are many of the concerns and problems surrounding the use of human subjects in research, bringing into conflict not only values but the very purposes and definitions of life itself. Implicit on every page is the increasing ground swell for the right to know why, where, and how participation in research will be determined. The persistent and salient message that emerges from a review of this record is that men and women of integrity and good will can differ in perspective and terminology while attempting with determination and no little anguish to find answers that will be acceptable to all segments of a democratic society. The Academy Forum was initiated to offer a public platform for such dialogue, and it will continue to address some of the hard and unanswered questions posed herein.

Robert R. White
Director

iv

CONTENTS

vi

DAY I

DAY I
AN OVERVIEW

Frederick C. Robbins
Chairman

This Forum was organized because of the great concern about human experimentation in this country today. The reasons for this concern are not all easy to identify, but they include a number of well-publicized real or imagined abuses, a subject which was not dealt with in any detail during the first day of this Forum. Many of the medical investigators who have spoken have indicated that abuses are rare, whereas other participants have implied that they suspect that they are quite common. However, no substantial documentation has been provided by either side, nor has there been any discussion of specific cases except for the hypothetical one of the panel on children. Undoubtedly the level of concern is heightened by the discussion of many actual and imagined advances in science and technology with potential fearsome consequences such as genetic engineering, behavior modification, and organ transplantation. As pointed out by Dr. Renée Fox, important questions are being raised within our society concerning the rights of the individual as opposed to the needs of the community as a whole -- authority is being challenged generally, and this includes the medical profession, which to many has an authoritarian image. Although this may well be healthy for our society, and I am rather inclined to think it is, nonetheless it presents problems for many groups of people, including medical investigators.

During the day's discussion much was said about the benefits of biomedical research and the importance of human experimentation in bringing these benefits to pass. It was pointed out that no new treatment or procedure can be introduced without going through a period of trial and experimentation involving, eventually, trials in man. It was also pointed out that such trials cannot be done without a certain amount of risk -- and it is always necessary to judge, to the best of our ability, risks versus benefits. However, it is also clear that this not only applies to procedures that are developmental or experimental but also to many procedures that are considered established and about which questions of risk are no longer raised. It is important to keep in mind the distinction between experimentation that is therapeutically motivated and from which the subject is likely to benefit from that which is nontherapeutic or from which the subject cannot benefit. The information to be derived will be of benefit to others, possibly to the subject himself in the future.

The subject of therapeutic trials and the use of controls and/or placebos was not addressed in today's dicussion. In recent years, perhaps particularly triggered by the Kefauver hearings of some years ago, there has been great concern that drugs and other procedures be shown to be efficacious as well as safe before they are licensed for general use. It is difficult to quarrel with this point of view and generally it has received much support; however, it has an immediate consequence, namely that trials must be conducted not only in animals or in the laboratory but in man -- and not only in man but in man at the appropriate stage of development -- since the adult cannot be equated with the child, and the fetus presents unique problems.

A properly designed double blind trial means that there must be controls. The control is given an innocuous substance or a treatment that has been standard in the past or may receive a placebo that, again, is an innocuous substance presumably from which he will derive no benefit other than a psychological one. It is a major problem and one that those responsible for licensure of drugs and biologicals and those attempting to develop new therapeutic agents and procedures find most troublesome. Thus as we attempt on the one hand to pursue the highly laudable goal of demonstrating efficacy of those things we do, we immediately find ourselves presented with the ethical problems involved in large-scale trials in man.

The issue of informed consent presented our speakers and participants serious problems. In general, informed consent was regarded as a keystone of ethical human experimentation. However, as was pointed out on a number of occasions, truly informed consent is a difficult condition to arrive at; and, on some occasions, full disclosure of the details of an experiment may invalidate it. Nonetheless, it would seem that there was general agreement on the need for proper informed consent; but, above all, full disclosure of the details of the experiment and the risks and benefits to be derived. The degree to which the investigator himself should be solely responsible for the explanations and determining consent was a matter of some difference of opinion; but there was no difference of opinion about the fact that the procedures involved and the experiment itself should be subject to independent review, which is generally the case today in most institutions engaged in human experimentation.

As was foreseen in the design of the Forum, the problem of informed consent becomes moot when one is dealing with persons who cannot give appropriate consent, either because of their circumstances or because of their inability to understand. During this first day of the Forum, two special circumstances were discussed: namely, the problem of the fetus and the problem of the child.

Fetal research was difficult for the participants to deal with. The discussion largely centered around the need for fetal research and the benefits that have been and can be derived therefrom. Little was heard from those who oppose the use of the fetus. The relationship of fetal research to abortion was brought up, and one discussant suggested that they could and should be separated. However, in view of what has happened in a number of states in regard to legal restrictions on fetal research, it is hard to believe that concern about abortion is not a key factor that makes it difficult to discuss the issue in rational terms. Assuming that fetal research is to be done, who can give permission? Informed consent, in this instance, cannot be obtained from the subject; and under circumstances of planned abortion where the mother, and often father as well, have made the decision to terminate a pregnancy, their right to give permission or to make disposition of the fetus seems highly compromised in the minds of many people.

The possibility that fetal tissues might be marketed commercially or that the decision to have an abortion might be influenced by the possibility of gain was raised and appeared to be a new thought to most of the participants. Whether or not a previable fetus should be treated in the same way as a potentially viable fetus is a controversial matter. Whether or not the previable fetus is considered to be a person or the equivalent of a maternal organ has considerable to do with the kinds of experimentation that would be regarded as acceptable on the previable fetus. Unfortunately, it is not easy to define viability in absolute terms. Any arbitrary definition must be subject to revision, since with our improvements in technology younger and younger fetuses can be saved.

Another distinction of importance is between living and dead fetuses, since it is primarily experiments on "living" fetuses that are deplored. The definition of *living* in the case of a previable fetus is not easy to make, since once the fetus is separated from its life-support system, the mother, it is no longer an independent organism capable of sustaining itself. It was not made clear during the formal discussion that much of the important research cited does not require a living fetus. The experiments are done with bits of tissue or cells that can be secured in much the same way as organs or tissues are obtained at autopsy from older individuals. Relatively few experiments are done with what could be called, by any definition of which I am aware, a living fetus. Such experiments do present special emotional, and perhaps even ethical, problems; but only this way can certain kinds of information necessary to learn about the metabolism of the fetus at different stages in its development be obtained.

Can one justify doing anything in anticipation of abortion? This question arises because of the need to understand the effect upon the fetus of certain drugs, vaccines, or other environmental alterations. An example of such an experiment is the testing of an antibiotic or drug to determine whether or not it reaches the fetus, and, if it does, whether or not it is in any way injurious. Since, even after exhaustive testing in animals, it is often not possible to be certain that a procedure will be innocuous for the human fetus, most such experiments can only be done when the fetus did not survive. A special consideration is that the mother might change her mind when it is too late to reverse the procedure. In practice this does not seem to have been a problem. The British have adopted the position that only under very special circumstances can anything be done in anticipation of abortion.

In spite of its controversial nature, it does not seem that the extreme position that no research under any circumstances can be done on fetuses is in the best interests of society. It is not easy, however, to arrive at any compromise position. The distinction between research on living fetuses and dead fetuses might allow for some compromise, namely restricting research on living, as opposed to dead, fetuses. It is unlikely that a position will ever be arrived at that will be satisfactory to those persons who are opposed to abortion under any circumstances, since the fetal research-abortion issues seem firmly linked in their minds. Nonetheless, the approach taken by the British, in which an arbitrary statement, subject to revision, of the criteria for viability were made and certain very specific guidelines were laid down that limit, but do not prohibit, fetal research is a reasonable approach.

In considering the peculiar problems of research on children, it was pointed out that it is important to do some research on children, since they differ from adults in their response to drugs and other procedures. However, concern was expressed about doing any research on children that was not of direct benefit to the subject. Indeed, it was suggested that parents do not have or should not have the right to give permission for participation of their children in such experiments. The proposal that all children more than seven years of age should be asked to give consent before participation in experiments provoked disagreement, since it was felt that children so young would be unable to comprehend the circumstances and to give truly informed consent. The age at which this could reasonably be expected was not agreed upon; and, indeed, the differences in rates of maturation among individual children make it difficult to draw an arbitrary line. However, somewhere between the ages of twelve and sixteen seemed to be reasonable in the opinion of certain of the participants. The problem of institutionalized children is an even more difficult one and here, again, a serious question was raised as to whether or not anyone has the right to give permission for such children to participate in research.

It was obvious during the entire discussion that the mechanisms that we now have for obtaining consent for those who cannot give it for themselves -- this includes children, the fetus, institutionalized children, and the mentally retarded -- are probably inadequate. Some better mechanism must be developed, whether it is through the courts or by some more innovative method; there seems to be a need to provide a responsible surrogate who can protect the interests of these individuals. Traditionally, where available, a responsible family should be able to do this with proper guidance and support. Unfortunately, not all families are responsible; and, therefore, even when there is a family some assessment of their capability to preserve their child's best interests is desirable.

The effectiveness of the present review mechanism for human experimentation was a matter of much interest. All institutions that conduct research with federal funding are required to have a committee that is responsible for review of all proposed experimentation involving humans; and not only must they approve the project before it is initiated, but they also have responsibility for continued monitoring of the project. Although limited, the discussion revealed that there is concern about the composition of these committees. In general, it seemed that most agreed that, in order to have a proper review of the ethical concerns, the medical investigators should be assisted by nonmedical persons. However, as yet there seems to be no complete agreement as to the proper number and kinds of such persons to be included on the committees. A question was raised concerning the degree to which the actions of the committees were made public and the kinds of records that are kept. Mr. Halperin proposed that the entire review process should be subject to investigation to find out what is going on around the country, how satisfactorily the procedures are being followed, and what might be done to improve the process. Indeed, he suggested that the entire subject of experimentation with man should be approached in an experimental way.

A final matter that was raised was that of providing some type of indemnification of the subjects of research in case of injury or loss as the result of experimentation. This seems like a subject that is amenable to solution once it is agreed that it is the proper thing to do.

It would seem reasonable to conclude that:

1. The concern about the way in which human experimentation is conducted is greater than many investigators realize.

2. It is not enough to calculate risk-benefit ratios, but ethical, moral, and political considerations must be taken into account as well. However, it seems not to be generally recognized that the movement towards demanding proof of efficacy of the therapeutic measures implies greater need for experimentation involving man.

3. Although informed consent is a critical requirement for the ethical conduct of research, new means need to be created to provide a surrogate to serve those subjects who cannot give informed consent for themselves.

4. The appropriate conduct of research on humans should be addressed as a suitable subject for critical research.

WELCOME

Philip Handler
President
National Academy of Sciences

My purpose here is to welcome you to the National Academy of Sciences. This is the third of a series of forums and a new and experimental mode by which the Academy hopes to be of service.

About two years ago, we decided that there is required, somewhere, a platform for discussion and debate of controversial issues of public policy concerning matters that involve a considerable degree of technical content. Successful organization of such a forum is not easy. It reminds me of the house I owned in North Carolina. Immediately around the house was a small lawn, surrounded by several acres of woodland. Many of our visitors would note how pleasantly natural the woods looked and would offer sympathy that the lawn had to be mowed. The reality was that the lawn could be mowed in fifteen minutes, but it was back-breaking work to keep those woods looking "natural."

Similarly, to excite interest and conflict sufficient to arouse what we hope will be heated, natural, uninhibited debate when the floor will be yours, we have planned, in detail, presentations by speakers of differing views, who, however, may or may not contradict each other. When the positions are truly polarized, such debates give rise to more heat than light. The opponents usually talk past each other rather than at each other. Nevertheless, in our previous forums we have had a few moments when there was real confrontation and enough light was shed so that the others in the room understood the real differences and were able to make evaluative judgments of their own. That is the purpose of these exercises.

The subject of the present Forum is very much in the national eye and has elicited much interest from all quarters of our society. The problem itself, however, is by no means new; it has been with us since the beginnings of experimental medicine. It is not likely to be resolved in these two days; but if we emerge with a better understanding, then our purpose will have been served.

Many in this room have had personal encounters with diverse facets of the problem of using human subjects in experimentation. I have a list of my own. There was the time when I was among the first normal controls to swallow nicotinic acid. I had no thought of being at risk, but, at dinner that evening, I suddenly felt as if a Bunsen flame was being played upon my back. Thus was the vasodilatory property of nicotinic acid discovered. Happily, that is all it did; it might have done more. Such an experiment would be undertaken with much more caution today. But what should one think of the fact that this somewhat useful property of nicotinic acid would not have been nearly so readily discovered with animal subjects?

Another time that I recall vividly was when two medical students and I were engaged in studying the response to intravenously administered parathyroid hormone. Unbeknowst to us, until that time no one had ever been given parathyroid hormone who was not recumbent. We gave each other the extract intravenously and went about our business in the laboratory, preparing for the analyses we were to undertake. Suddenly, all three of us were on the floor. Thus was first observed the fall in blood pressure that follows the injection of parathyroid extract. Again, happily, that turned out without serious consequence. But there were some very bad moments.

Those risks are ancient risks. Given the ultimate need to know how a potentially useful drug affects a normal individual, some degree of untoward events is inevitable. What frequency is to be deemed acceptable? Rather early on in the history of transplantation antigens, when tissue typing had just become practicable, it was proposed at our medical school that all the inmates in a nearby prison be thus typed, in the hope that they might be identified as potential kidney donors. The prison authorities had already agreed when the proposal was brought to the executive committee of our medical faculty. Two of us were adamant in insisting that this not be done unless all of our faculty and medical students also were willing to participate. An individual who chanced to match the tissue type of a needy recipient would be subject to a kind of moral suasion which is difficult to resist; to have picked that particular population seemed to us to be inappropriate and unwarranted. The program was not implemented. Whether anyone later was deprived of life-rendering assistance as a result of that decision, I will never know.

Some of the problems of weighing the risks versus the benefits of the conduct of research using human subjects will be put before you this morning and then illuminated during the course of the rest of the meeting. These problems, as we have seen, are not new. But our sensibilities have been heightened in recent years, and it is because of this heightening that it seems imperative that we reexamine this old subject in an attempt to help our country frame policy in these regards. As you know, a Commission has been appointed to attend to that task; that Commission, like ourselves, will require education.

Most of the medical schools and teaching hospitals in the United States have come a long way in their behavior in these matters. It is no longer possible for an isolated investigator to go off on his own and simply do as he pleases. He is now accountable to his colleagues, in advance, before he may undertake any proposed experiment. Indeed, that very process has increased the sophistication of current medical research. However, few of us think that current procedures for accountability are adequate and sufficient for our societal purposes. It is in the hope of getting a step closer to what such procedures should be in the future that this Forum has been convened. I hope that, by tomorrow afternoon, all of us will have significantly more insight than we do this morning.

PERSPECTIVES
OF BIOMEDICAL
RESEARCH

A CULTURAL AND HISTORICAL VIEW

Francis D. Moore

INTRODUCTION

Human experimentation is a daily occurrence in the practice of medicine
because of the uniqueness of the individual. Whether it be the first
dose of insulin in a diabetic or of digitalis in the cardiac, the method
of careful planning based on a background of knowledge, with honest evaluation of results, plays a key role.

Every surgical operation is an experiment in bacteriology. It is
also an experiment in the pharmacology of anesthetic drugs (the only
drugs that we regularly use to take patients into deep coma), in the
conformity to anatomical norms, and often in the biology of malignant
tumors. It is far better to recognize these uncertainties and the
insecurity of the individual in a sea of statistical probability, than
it is to move the other way and to routinize medical care under the
delusion that all people are the same. It is the very application of
the scientific experimental method to medicine that permits an ethical
outcome in the endless variety of human disease and the unpredictable
patterns of emotional response.

Although this basic experimental nature of clinical medicine and,
indeed, of all human intercourse is not the subject of this Forum, it
is an essential and appropriate introduction because experimental observation in man displays a continuum or a spectrum that starts at the
bedside. This spectrum stretches from the daily uncertainties of drugs
and procedures to several much more difficult areas.

The most familiar of these more troublesome areas is that of therapeutic innovation. Whether it be the first trial of new drugs, of
vaccines, or of surgical procedures, there must always be a "first",
and this is *always* human experimentation. Beyond these clinical trials

15

is the area of experimentation in patients who *might* profit from the knowledge gained (often at some unspecified, later time), sort of a general humane promise. This is the basis for much of "clinical investigation."

Finally, we come to experimentation in persons not expected thereby to benefit at all, persons possibly hurt and hurt badly (or their lives endangered) when they wittingly or unwittingly provide the body of a sentient, erect-walking biped for biological experimentation. From this last area of experimentation have come some of the glories of medicine and of public health: the conquest of yellow fever, the rout of typhus, the perfection of blood transfusion and, most recently, space travel, surely a most remarkable form of human experimentation. Experience suggests that our intuitive judgments on all these are partly based on retrospective outcome analysis, surely a weak reed to lean on in the ethical jungle. From this last form of experimentation come also some of the darkest chapters and some of the most flagrant abuses of the societal privilege of physicians and scientists.

In focusing some historical perspectives as an introduction to this Forum, I should point out that it is not a new field. I refer you to the translation of the Smith Papyrus (c.2500 B.C.). That earliest recorded experience of man in treating illness clearly shows the insecurity, the uncertainty, and the essentially experimental method of medicine.

It is my intent here to explore the spectrum just mentioned and to review a few historical examples that demonstrate the folly of general or abstract rules, and the hazards of hasty judgment.

I am going to tell of each case briefly and try to analyze some of the salient features of each as examples of bold, sometimes hazardous, and not always successful experiments in man.

Smallpox - 1721

I would like to begin by going back 250 years to the first example of public health and epidemiology conducted in North America.

About 1718, the Reverend Cotton Mather, who was only a few short years from the witch burnings, learned of African natives who recognized that the scars of smallpox meant that one would never have the disease again; they occasionally and purposely gave each other the disease. Lady Montague, wife of the British Ambassador to Constantinople, also had known that the Turks did this. Because Mather was a corresponding member of the Royal Society, he had become aware of this information.

Although Boston was repeatedly ravaged by lethal smallpox epidemics, Mather could not find any local doctors willing to undertake this dangerous and innovative procedure. So he turned to a small nearby community known as "Muddy River" -- now Brookline. There he found Dr. Zabdiel Boylston, who was the son of a doctor but had no medical degree of his own. Mather talked him into it, and Boylston went ahead with the experiment. He did not inoculate himself because he had already had the disease; even though there was no word for immunity, he knew what it meant. Boylston started with his child. The boy developed what was called a "discrete" case (which means that each pock was separate) was sick for a few days, and got well.

Boylston went on to inoculate a great many other people. This was inoculation with the virus of smallpox; this was not vaccination with the virus of cowpox.

The following illustrations are taken from Boylston's book[1] on this hazardous exercise in human experimentation.

In Figure 1 is shown the title page of the 1726 corrected second edition of *An Historical Account of the Small-Pox Inoculated in New England,* originally published in London. It was further published in Boston in 1730. The comprehensiveness of its contents as well as the dedication bear notice.

Figure 2 is a sample page that gives a clear indication of the scope of Boylston's carefully detailed work and the nature of his observations.

Historical A C C O U N T

OF THE

S M A L L - P O X

I N O C U L A T E D

IN

NEW ENGLAND,

Upon all Sorts of Perfons, *Whites, Blacks,* and of all Ages and Conftitutions.

With fome Account of the Nature of the Infection in the NATURAL and INOCULATED Way, and their different Effects on HUMAN BODIES.

With fome fhort DIRECTIONS to the UN-EXPERIENCED in this Method of Practice.

Humbly dedicated to her Royal Highnefs the Princefs of WALES,

By *Zabdiel Boylston,* F. R. S.

The Second Edition, Corrected.

L O N D O N:

Printed for S. CHANDLER, at the Crofs-Keys in the Poultry. M. DCC. XXVI.

Re-Printed at *B O S T O N* in *N. E.* for S. GERRISH in *Cornhil,* and T. HANCOCK at the Bible and Three Crowns in *Annftreet.* M. DCC. XXX.

FIGURE 1

(11)

fhould take it in the natural way, fhe fuffer'd me to make the proper Incifions; after which at the 7th Day, her Fever came on, and the Small Pox came out on the 9th pretty full of the diftinct Sort: She had fomething more of a Fever than is ufual this way, and about the height of the Diftemper her *Menfes* came down, which added to her Uneafineffes a few Days; but all went over, and fhe foon got well. It was ftrongly reported, that fhe mifcarry'd; but upon ftrict Inquiry of the Nurfe, I found it falfe and groundlefs, fhe not being then with Child.

I inoculated Mrs. *Dodge,* about 20 Years old, who had nurfed her Sifter, then lying fick of the Confluent Small-Pox, until the 7th Day from her Eruption: She being terrify'd with the Circumftances of her Sifter, I was perfuaded by her Mother and felf to inoculate her, which I did, by way of Experiment: She had the Small-Pox at the ufual Time, with very little Sicknefs or Pain, and fcarce an hundred in all: She was fo foon well, it could hardly be faid fhe had been fick.

5th, I inoculated Juftice *Lynde's* Negro Boy, about 17 Years old, he had the Small-Pox at the ufual Time, and of a very kind diftinct Sort, and foon was well.

6th, I inoculated my three Daughters, *Jerufha* of about 10, *Mary* 8, and *Elizabeth* 4 Years old; the eldeft had but about 40 or 50, the other two were pretty full in their Faces; and all their Symptoms proving gentle, they foon did well.

7th, I inoculated Mr. *Elias Adams,* about 18 Years of Age, he had the Small-Pox at the com-
D 2   mon

FIGURE 2

Further on in the book we find this table (Figure 3) citing the number of persons inoculated as well as the names and dates of ensuing deaths. Here, in this first recorded study of any attempt to deal with public health in America, we find detailed data (Figure 4). Of the 286 people inoculated, including thirty-nine from Roxbury and Cambridge, there were six deaths. Boylston recognized, as he notes, that some of these may have been "infected in the natural Way, before Inoculated." Lastly in Figure 5 we have here a statement that clearly implies the success of Boylston's work. In 1721 and early 1722, Boston was ravaged by another smallpox epidemic: 5,759 persons had the disease naturally, culminating in 844 deaths. Comparing these numbers with Boylston's indicates that individuals receiving his inoculations experienced about a 2-percent mortality, while the natural disease produced a 15-percent mortality.

This hazardous experiment, which was carried out with very little background and the most primitive knowledge, paved the way for

(50)

not, in Time, inoculated them again, and so prevented that Misfortune.

In case you should have, thro' ill Habits of Body, or the like, any of your Inoculations that will not give way to, and heal with white Bread and Milk, treat them as you would do other common Sores, viz. with Fomentations and stronger Digestives, &c.

A TABLE shewing the Number Inoculated by me in each Month in the Year 1721 & 1722. with the ill Success attending the same, viz. Who dyed and When.

June	3	0
July	7	0
August	17	1
Septemb.	31	0	Mrs. Dixwell September 24th.
October	18	0	Mr. Dorr's Indian Girl December 9th.
November	103	2	John White Esq; December 10th.
December	50	3	Mrs. Bethiah Scarborough, December 11th.
January	7	0	Mrs. Wells, December 18th.
February	5	0	Mrs. Serle, January 3d.
March		
April		
May	6	0
	247	6

FRom my Experience in them that liv'd as well as those 5 who died in the Cold Weather, I would advise those who are weak and infirm, that may come into this practice, and that live in a cold Country, to avoid November, December, & January, for I have reason to believe that if Mrs. Wells, Serle, Scarborough, and the Indian Girl, had been Inoculated in a temperate or warmer Season, they wou'd have done well. And it may be worthy of Note, that in above One Hundred and Fifty Males, that were Inoculated here, and of which Number Eighty odd were Men, but only one died. APPEN-

FIGURE 3

(34)

Their Ages.	Persons inoculated.	Had a perfect Small-Pox by Inoculation.	Had an Imperfect Small-Pox.	Had no Effect.	Suspected to have died of Inoculation.
From 9 Mon. to 2 years old	07	07	00	00	00
2 to 5	14	14	00	00	00
5 to 10	16	16	00	00	00
10 to 15	29	29	00	00	00
15 to 20	48	47	01	00	01
20 to 30	67	65	00	02	01
30 to 40	44	42	00	02	01
40 to 50	08	07	00	01	00
50 to 60	07	06	00	01	02
60 to 67	07	07	00	00	01
Total	247	242	01	06	06
Inoculated by Drs Roby and Thompson in Roxbury and Cambridge	39	39	00	00	00
Total	286	281	01	06	06

It appears by the foregoing Table, that Inoculation upon six Persons did not produce the Small-Pox, by Reason they had had it before. And that out of 286, six died, though they had not all the Small-Pox only by Inoculation, as we have Reason to believe, but were some of them infected in the natural Way, before Inoculated. And it further appears by our Practice in New-England, that if a Number of Per-

FIGURE 4

(33)

pinion of this ; and until then, I fhall value and
efteem this Method of inoculating the Small-
Pox, as the moft beneficial and fuccefsful that
ever was difcover'd to, and practifed by Mankind in this World.

In the Year 1721, and Beginning of 1722.
there were, in *Bofton*, 5759 Perfons who had
the Small-Pox in the natural Way, out of which
Number died 844, (this Account I took from
one of our Prints, publifhed by Authority) fo
that the Proportion that died of the naturalSmall
Pox there, appears to be one in fix, or between
that of fix & feven.

The following Table will fhew the Difference
between the Succefs of the natural Small-Pox,
and that of the inoculated, in *New-England*.

FIGURE 5

seventy-five years of some -- however uncertain -- protection against
epidemic smallpox. The inoculation was used by General Washington in
the Revolutionary Army. Boylston, originally ridiculed and scorned,
lived to receive honor and vindication both here and abroad. He paved
the way for the acceptance in this country of Jenner's great contribution of cowpox vaccination when Benjamin Waterhouse brought it from
England.

Looking back, what is interesting about all this? First, the doctor
was persuaded by a man of the church! Second, the procedure was undertaken with no preliminary animal work whatsoever. It was based largely
on hearsay and the universal observation that if you had the scar you
had the badge of immunity.* It should also be recognized that a mortality of 2 percent would be absolutely unacceptable in any present-day
review of human experimentation. But it led to protection and opened
the door for future work.

---

*Please note -- for the example 250 years later -- that if you had the
characteristic flaccid paralysis you never got polio again!

Polio - 1934

Our second example, advancing along the spectrum, moves forward two centuries to the polio immunization trials in the middle 1930s. Starting in about 1932, Dr. Brodie and Dr. Park of New York had grown some polio virus in monkey spinal cord, which they had then inactivated with formalin. On the basis of about twenty monkeys, they inoculated about three thousand children. At the same time, John Kolmer of Philadelphia, working with a rather different virus preparation, inoculated himself and then his children. On the basis of forty-two monkeys, he then did a very large experiment, the exact numbers of which were never recorded.

Dr. John Paul, in his *History of Poliomyelitis*,[2] states that Brodie's results constituted evidence that immunity could be developed against the polio virus by using a virus rendered noninfective by formalin. This finding, as it turned out in later years, was of major significance and not far off the mark. But Brodie acted on it far too precipitously by rushing into human use. His haste was attributable in part to his desire to be ahead of his competitor. Otherwise Brodie would not have taken the risks he did by barging into a program involving the immunization of so many children with a vaccine that had been tried on only about twenty monkeys. Within the first year there were several cases of polio from these two experiments. Some of them resulted in paralysis and some in death. And what of the scientist? Paul gives this account:

> To poor Brodie, on the other hand, failure was a crushing blow. During the early days of his experimental work everything seemed to be going well. He had received many flattering offers, but after 1935, such offers ceased abruptly, and Brodie was hard put to find a place to work. Eventually he accepted a minor position. He died shortly later. It is alleged that he took his own life, a tragic end for one who started out with such high hopes.

The startling thing about this story -- and this is an important consideration -- was the impact that a poorly conceived experiment had on the entire field. Paul sums this up as follows: "The events of 1935 cut more deeply into progress in the immunization of man against poliomyelitis than most people realized at the time." He tells of a meeting held in 1946 by the National Foundation for Infantile Paralysis, then active, at which a report was given by Dr. Morgan of Johns Hopkins on immunization progress in monkeys. One of the participants at the meeting said, "The time has come to find out what happens in man: to study his immune reactions, and to get on with new attempts to produce evidence of artificial immunity in man." At this, according to Paul, "a veritable shudder went round the room."

The responsibility of the scientist is not only to his subjects, not only to his science, but he may, unwittingly, have an effect on the whole subsequent development of the field.

Polio - 1960

Our third example is the successful development of polio vaccine. Since John Enders long has been a friend of mine and I have made a hobby of considering the various aspects of his work, it is a particular and re- markable pleasure to discuss that work in the presence of today's chair- man, Dr. Robbins, one of the major contributors to the great discovery.

Most of you know the story, but there are several features that are very important. First, youth was involved: two young men, one of them starting as a medical student, working with a senior scientist. It was a group endeavor with constant open review and publication: beware of the single man who wants to keep his work secret. Cautious interpreta- tion was characteristic throughout. Human fetal tissue[3] was the basic breakthrough, as described so clearly by Dr. Enders in his Nobel address. The placebo was critically important: the initial plan involved 30,000 children who would receive a false injection. One could be certain that some of those children would get polio, and some would die.

It also is interesting that it encountered serious trouble at one point with the so-called "Cutter incident," an example of a scientific (viral) aspect more complicated than a commercial process could master. But the vaccine did have to be tried for the first time in man, in per- fectly well young children, with no therapeutic benefit -- only the promise of future prophylaxis in case they became exposed. Some who were to receive the placebo, as I have said, were sure to be exposed, and some would get the disease.

Figure 6 shows the trio of Nobel laureates that produced the polio vaccine. From left to right: Thomas H. Weller, John F. Enders, and Frederick C. Robbins.

Figure 7 shows a chart demonstrating the effect of the vaccine on the incidence of poliomyelitis, surely one of the most exciting achieve- ments of medicine in our generation.

Measles - 1962

Our fourth example also has to do with viruses and vaccines: the trial of attenuated measles vaccine in Africa. The knowledge that came from Africa to prompt Boylston's smallpox inoculations in 1721 has now been taken back in several ways. I mention it briefly, but it brings up an interesting point. In the first page of the Katz article it says, "In the United States of America, we had acquired little experience with the use of the Edmonston vaccine in malnourished children. That was some- thing that needed to be done. With this background and with an aware- ness of the problems generated by measles in Nigeria, we felt justified in undertaking a careful study of attenuated virus vaccine amongst Yoruba children."[4] So this was basically an experiment to acquire new knowledge.

22

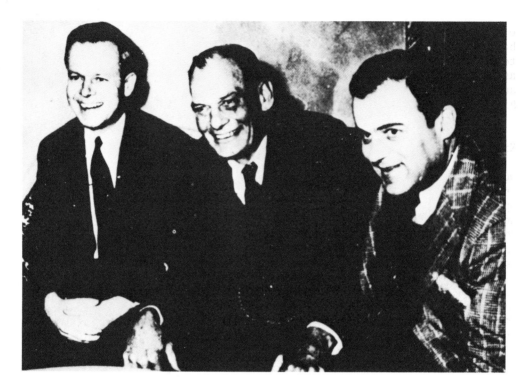

FIGURE 6

ANNUAL POLIOMYELITIS INCIDENCE RATES
UNITED STATES, 1935-1964

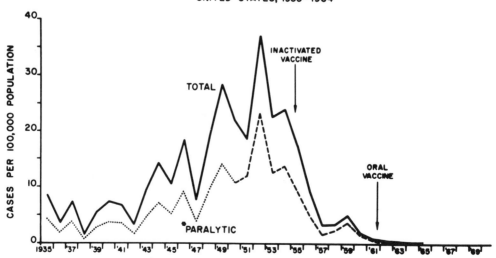

FIGURE 7

There are many aspects there, but the most interesting is the problem of informed consent. There is no way across that language and cultural barrier that this procedure could ever be adequately explained either to the child or to the mother in an African jungle tribe. The results, as you know, were impressive. Measles, a plague of that part of Nigeria and Upper Volta, was wiped out, and those who did this were given the highest honor of that same African tribe. Informed consent?

Kidney Transplant - 1950

Our fifth example is that of kidney transplantation, and it has two interesting subsets. The first was the work by Willem Kolff in developing the artificial kidney, which he did in 1941 and 1942 in Holland under the eyes of the Nazis, who were absolutely unaware of what he was doing. He had known of the previous work in 1915 at Johns Hopkins showing the passage through a dialysis membrane of many of the small molecules that make people sick with renal failure.

He also was aware of the work in 1938 of McEwen in Chicago, who tried to set this type of thing up with collodion membranes. Kolff had some sausage casing and a tomato can. From these he made a primitive artificial kidney.[5] In 1962, when I was writing a little history of this, I corresponded with Dr. Kolff. In his reply he said that it was an awfully good thing that he did not do that work in a particularly well-organized department of medicine where there were a lot of rules, because all of his first patients died. They died, of course, of renal failure that he could not reverse, but he did show that the biochemical and clinical manifestations were reversible. His work established a new method and laid the groundwork for transplantation.

In 1951 and 1952, the late Dr. Hume, working with Dr. Thorn and Dr. Dammin, carried out nine kidney transplatations in unmodified recipients, working out the anatomy and where to place the kidney -- not in the leg, but in the belly -- and how to hook it up. They found that the patient was soon up and around, feeling fine. All the transplants failed. All the patients died. It was a remarkable therapeutic attempt. It would be impossible to get this by any of the so-called "Human Use Committees" at the present time.

Figure 8 shows a picture that Dr. Kolff took in Holland of the four kidneys that he had made. He left one there and took one to Britain, where it was enshrined in St. Bartholomew's Hospital. He took one to Russia, and said that he never heard of it again. Dr. George Thorn and Dr. Carl Walter obtained the fourth one and made from it their new variation of the kidney which, as you know, looked very much like this for many years.

What are some of the interesting aspects of this? First, they were all transplants of cadaver kidneys. We felt, at that stage, it was unwise to use a living donor. These experiences showed clearly that all the clinical physiological and psychological manifestations of renal failure were reversible. If the patient's sick kidneys were taken out,

24

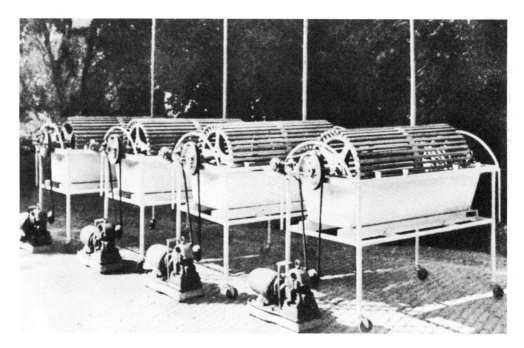

FIGURE 8

the blood pressure came down, and it set the stage for what was to happen quite unexpectedly just eighteen months later when the first identical twin pair showed up. When they came along it was perfectly clear how to do the operation to have prolonged success.

It is interesting that one of those patients of the first nine lived for 180 days. He went back to South America and resumed his practice of medicine. Later, when he was in his terminal illness, having rejected the kidney, his only words were those of thanks to the very hardworking team of many people -- doctors, nurses, and all their helpers -- who had given him some hope at the end.

These trials gave hope to lots of people. In that same year Billingham, Brent, and Medewar published their paper on acquired tolerance. In 1960, 6-MP and azathioprine came along, and at least a temporary way of helping people with renal failure became available: transplantation under immunosuppresion.

It often seems strange that many patients, especially with severe organ disease (such as liver failure or kidney failure, or with malignant tumors) come to physicians *specifically asking that new and untried things be attempted*. They will go to another doctor or another hospital if they are not assured of such trials. Much has been made of the human guinea pig. Patients come to us and *ask* to be one. *They want to try the untried because they know that the tried has always failed.*

Frequently they want to give a favorable judgment on the trial, and therein lies a trap for the unwary.

Krebiozen - 1955

It is this very desire of the sick patient to say that he or she is better that has lead many an investigator down the primrose path. This was true for Dr. Andrew C. Ivy and "Krebiozen." For further details of that unfortunate saga and of how the wish of patients to be helped can lead an investigator astray, I refer you to the Boylston Society Essay of Dr. William D. Morain, "Krebiozen: Nineteen Years of Controversy"[6] and to my account in *Daedalus*.[7] Suffice it to say here that this was one of the sorriest episodes in American science: the promotion of a secret nostrum by a formerly eminent physiologist.

Starvation - 1942

My final example is in many ways the most remarkable. It comes from the Warsaw Ghetto in 1942. The Germans were forcing the Jewish people into a very small area. A part of Warsaw that normally held 60,000 people had an unsupportable population of 1.5 million at its peak. About 50,000 a year died, for the Germans had learned that density of population hastened death. Young adults fit for forced labor were fed and used, pitted against the young and the old who were starved to death. Starvation, therefore, was extreme, and many died of it.

To study the dynamics of human starvation under these conditions of misery would seem the most inhumane sort of Nazi crime -- as bad as immersing political prisoners in ice cold water to see how long downed aviators could live in the Arctic.

A book was then written on the nature of this starvation.[8] There are only one or two copies in the United States. I am indebted to Dr. Jan Dmochowski for translating it and for helping me to understand it. This book describes the process of enforced mass starvation.

When we look at the list of authors, our hasty ethical judgment is turned completely around: all were Jewish physicians, and all but one died either in the Warsaw Ghetto uprising or in the gas chambers. The one who did live was Dr. Apfelbaum, whose son is now a distinguished nutritionist.

These doctors were trying to create something of lasting worth from the hopeless misery of their people. Here is one quotation:

> Our persecutors were using all possible methods to degrade us as human beings. They wanted to prove that we were a subhuman race. One of the methods used was starvation. When this was not quick enough, other methods were used. There were those of us who were trained and educated to conduct scientific studies, and we felt that this was a form of defiance that would be most appropriate

26

for us. From amongst several individuals participating in this study, almost no one survived. Their last work was left as a legacy for future generations of physicians.

Figure 9 shows the title page of the book, a copy of which is in the National Medical Library. It reads starkly and simply, *Starvation Disease*.

Figure 10 shows the wasting, the sort of starvation the physicians were observing. They carefully recorded the findings on autopsy, the nature of death; they did everything they could to try to understand what was going on.

The title of Figure 11 is "Forced Relocation." What you see here was the result of persistent constriction of the ghetto area. The ghetto experience, then, is an example where the question of *who performed the study* becomes critical in ethical judgment.

At the outset I said that judgments in this area are made partly on the basis of outcome (which seems unfortunate and Machiavellian) and partly in the context of the prevailing ethical climate that grows out of common knowledge and judgment. There are few absolutes. The Warsaw

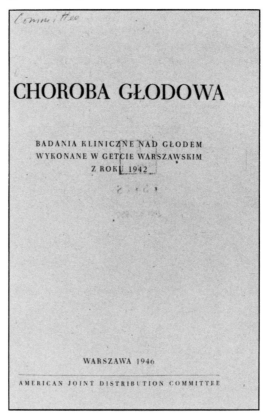

FIGURE 9

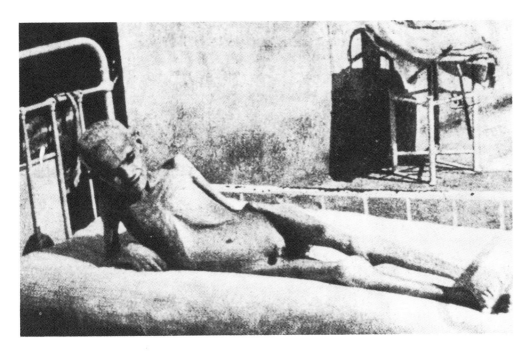

FIGURE 10

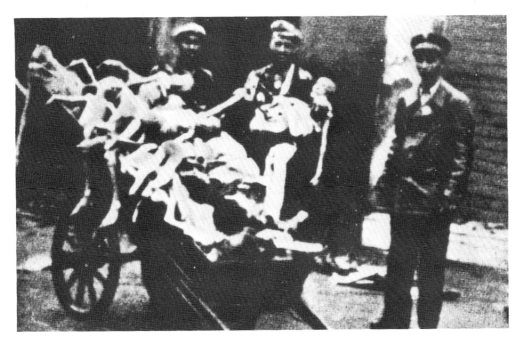

FIGURE 11

Ghetto example is one in which everything about it makes one of the truly dreadful stories of our years, except for these efforts of physicians to bring something worthwhile out of it.

Ethical Guidelines for Human Experimentation

Are there guidelines or general statements one can make? Is this a field wherein there should be a rigid set of federal regulations? We seem to have a great American genius for identifying a social problem and then trying to solve it by federal regulation; I give you the Eighteenth Amendment to the Constitution as an example. We must remind ourselves that it is not always necessary to solve problems by federal regulation!

Let me briefly review a checklist of components and characteristics that have proven vital to the ethics, integrity, and efficacy of biomedical research carried out in man. These components relate to the institution, the academic process, open disclosure, the problem of informed consent, laboratory background, and freedom of scientific growth.

First, let us consider *the institution*. A great deal of human experimentation of all types is done in teaching hospitals. Most of these institutions have become extremely sensitive to the many issues involved, and they are accustomed to surrounding each episode with the maximum safeguards in terms of a watchful and sensitive resident staff, the collaboration of a critical attending staff, and the laboratory services backup, which is essential to safety. When we depart from this environment, one must proceed with great caution. The Armed Services, the Space Administration, and other governmental agencies are not accustomed to human experimentation in which the welfare of the subject is of first concern. Private hospitals, or health spas that are trying to promote some special new cure or drug, should be regarded with supicion. Large industrial firms, whether they be aircraft manufacturers or drug houses, though concerned with human safety, have a conflict of interest that is patently obvious; safeguards should be maximized. Whenever it is possible, a sophisticated teaching hospital with strong university associations should maintain overview of the work. Where new "cures" or treatments are being investigated, such overview is particularly important, because to the unsophisticated, the universal way to achieve success on the part of patients may be quite misleading.

The academic process, if maintained in the best of the western traditions, is fundamentally an ethical process. It involves discussion, inquiry, openness and the presence of the learner, usually a young person. The learner is also a questioner, and frequently a doubter. One of the reasons that university hospitals have established an ethical climate for therapeutic innovation and other types of human experimentation is the presence of the academic process firmly entrenched. "Good science is ethical science" because the scientific process in itself, with an adequate conceptual background and honest evaluation of results, is in essence an ethical judgmental method. The same can be said of the academic process; when properly pursued, it is basically ethical.

Some of the worst abuses of human experimentation have occurred in situations far removed from the teaching hospital, and far removed from the academic environment: there has been no opportunity for question, inquiry, doubting, no students, and no open discussion.

The role of personal ambition in the scientific process has often been acknowledged as a sort of "motor power" that activates many scientists. Personal ambition, rivalry, ambition for advancement and promotion, are all characteristic components of university life. They present a severe hazard in the area of human experimentation. It is personal ambition to be the "first or the best" (and possibly to keep it a little secret during development) that is responsible for abuse. Openness, freedom of discussion, and presence of young people act as a strong counterbalance to the unbridled ego.

Appropriate laboratory background is so obvious that it need not be belabored here. There are very few things that can be done in human experimentation that are not amenable to some sort of preliminary laboratory study, either in the test tube or in an animal model. Not only should the laboratory background be adequately carried out, but preferably by the same persons who are to do the human work. Above all, the individuals involved should have encyclopedic knowledge of the literature of the field.

The matter of *informed consent* will be given much attention in this particular Forum of the National Academy of Sciences. In a way, the term is a contradiction in itself; if an experiment is being done, it means that the outcome is unknown. Therefore, it is impossible for anybody to be informed about it. On the other hand, the need is clear for a complete explanation of what is being done and an explanation of the processes, the hazards, and the possibilities. If the subject is in coma, incompetent, mentally deficient, at the extremes of life, then some sort of familial and legal process must be encompassed. When this is all done, one must admit that it is not truly informed consent, but that there has been an informational transaction of maximum depth.

Finally, *freedom of scientific inquiry is essential*. It is the rare scientist who has not changed his plan or changed his direction; sometimes the experiment is changed in midstream because things look promising or hazards can be reduced. One of the faults of government-sponsored contract research has been the extreme rigidity of protocols and a desire to avoid any opportunity for short-term ad hoc decisions. This is a very dangerous atmosphere for human experimentation. Controlled clinical trial suffers from this defect of being overly planned or "stage-managed." Sometimes the use of a placebo is essential, but as I mentioned previously, the use of placebos in an early vaccine trial may condemn some children to death. Then, the placebo must be abandoned. Nobody can be wise enough to make such judgments in advance. Freedom to change the protocol (as experience is gained) is essential for the ethical climate of human experimentation.

Under no circumstances should ethical decisions be made apart from the biological realities and in some cases the individual patient. There could be nothing more unethical than critical judgment in this field made by persons who have not studied the biology of the field or the patient.

A principal burden of this discourse is that while acknowledging the hazards of human experimentation, a far worse situation would result from overprotection. Restrictive laws, federal regulations, federally approved guidelines made contingent for research funding -- a form of federal penalty that has become popular today -- or the restriction of biomedical science entirely to animal work would have a remarkable adverse effect on the advance of knowledge and practical clinical care.

It remains true now, as always, that the basic study of man is man himself. It is equally true that no law or system of laws can stop the work of evil people whose only motive is personal gain. Society must protect human beings against exploitation, but naive or sweeping protective laws will fail of their mission and may slow the progress so much needed by the sick and suffering of coming generations.

THE BENEFITS OF RESEARCH

Lewis Thomas

There are two conflicting, polarized views of modern medical science, and the conflict between them accounts for much of today's public doubt and confusion concerning the proper role of medicine in society.

One view is that medicine is a full-fledged, mature science, possessed of enormous power to influence, change, and modify not only human disease but the normal conditions of human biology. Under this view, medicine has already come its full distance as a useful kind of science, and with so many conquests of disease credited to its accomplishment, feeling its own strength, it is looking around for new worlds to conquer. This is a prospect to frighten anyone. Given this view, no wonder there is apprehension about the new kinds of meddling we may soon be up to, from transplanting heads to cloning prominent political luminaries. If this is really the power of modern medicine, what are the limits which society should now be setting to the deployment of such power? Behavior control, genetic engineering, cloning, transplantation, immortality, all the rest of the hazardous prospects formerly dealt with by science fiction now seem to be immediately at hand, and something to worry about for tonight's insomnia. This is one view of things at one pole, and if this is what you believe about medicine, you will want all the protection from it that the law can provide.

The other view is that medicine is not, in fact, a proper science in any real sense. It is a fumbling, blundering, totally empirical non-science, incapable of influencing very much, if any, of our genuine health problems, rather pretentious in the public stance it takes, undeserving of the public acclaim it occasionally receives, and even conceivably, when you get right down to it, not necessary for the well-being of mankind. If this is the view you take, then you want to be sure that such a science, or pseudoscience, is not turned loose to be

31

fiddling around with human health, and you want protection from it as well.

The truth lies, I think, somewhere in between these extremes. Perhaps it would be useful, at the outset of these proceedings, to take a cool measuring look at the real position of modern medicine among the sciences, with special attention to its current capacity to do things and also to its current areas of incapacity.

There is no doubt at all that medicine has come a certain distance. But when you look at the whole range of major human diseases -- the disorders that cause premature death or prolonged incapacitation in great numbers of people, in all parts of the earth -- the distance we have come is relatively a very small fraction of the total run ahead. Medicine is, in fact, a proper science for what it is obliged to cope with, but it is a very young science, really only at its very beginning.

That beginning, however, has been both impressive and encouraging for the future. It lies mainly in the field of infectious diseases. Thanks to some extremely good basic science in the fields of microbiology, virology, and immunology, beginning late in the nineteenth century and continuing through the first third of this century, the principal pathogens of infectious disease were identified and classified. Viral vaccines were developed and applied to the prevention of the major childhood contagions, and the groundwork was laid for the discovery of the antibiotics and chemotherapy.

It needs emphasizing that penicillin, and the other subsequent antibiotics, represented a logical step in the scientific development of this field; but this step would not have been possible without the knowledge of bacterial pathogens that had come out of the preceding five decades of fundamental science. Before penicillin and the sulfonamides could be useful substances, you had to know that there were such things as pneumococci, streptococci, staphylococci, and meningococci, and you needed to know in some detail what these microorganisms were capable of doing to human beings.

What happened as the result of this accumulated information was nothing less than a revolution in health care. Most people have forgotten that there was such a revolution, because it happened so long ago. It is remembered most sharply, I think, by those who lived through it, and especially the generation of doctors who came out of medical school in the late 1930s.

I was one of these, and I have total recall for the transformation. It began in 1937, which was the year of my internship at the Boston City Hospital. This was the year when sulfanilamide first became available in this country. At that time there was a huge wing of the Boston City Hospital, known as the South Department, into which were crowded several hundred patients, mostly children, with contagious bacterial infections. The place was filled to overflowing throughout most of the year, but in the late winter and early spring it was almost intolerable. Most of the cases were streptococcal diseases, predominantly scarlet fever, with mastoiditis, rheumatic fever and glomerulonephritis as the typical, commonplace sequelae. There were, also, whole wards filled with diptheria, whooping cough, and meningococcol meningitis. The cases of diphtheria could be treated with antitoxin, but the patients with strep-tococcal and meningococcal infections were simply nursed through their illnesses, and there was always a substantial mortality.

There was a special ward in the main building of the Boston City Hospital set aside for the isolation of patients with erysipelas. These were mostly elderly people and alcoholics, many of whom died from this form of streptococcal infection. Out on the general wards the commonest disease throughout the winter months was lobar pneumonia. There were so many cases of this disease that they were assigned to the interns in rotation, according to a carefully kept "pneumonia count." This was necessary to prevent any one house officer from being overloaded and incapacitated by too many cases. If you had more than two or three new cases of lobar pneumonia to admit in a single night, you would expect to be without sleep for the next twenty-four hours or longer. Each case required the most intensive kind of nursing and supportive care. There were type-specific antipneumococcal sera available, and if you were lucky you could induce a crisis and bring the disease to an abrupt end in a few hours, but this technology was complex, chancy, and some-times dangerous. Typically, on a winter's night, there would be enough new cases of pneumonia to require the laying down of cots in the center of each of the hospital wards, and often these cots were lined up all the way out into the corridors and up to the elevator doors. My memo-ries of the City Hospital medicine of those days are all memories of bacterial infection, crowded beyond belief, mostly untreatable, and entirely unpreventable.

Then the sulfonamides arrived, and a few years later penicillin, and after that the rest of today's antibiotics. By the early 1950s the wards of the Boston City Hospital, and of all the other big city hospi-tals in this country, had begun to empty, and they have remained partly empty ever since. This change, which amounted to a revolution in itself, was not due to any change in the economics of health care. The patients had not gone off to other, more harmonious hospitals for their treatment. The diseases had themselves vanished. Lobar pneumonia became a rare disease. Scarlet fever and the complications of strepto-coccal infection became rarities. Pertussis and diphtheria vanished. Erysipelas vanished. Today, if a case of classical, clinically typical pneumonia is encountered in a large teaching hospital, the medical students are hailed in to see the phenomenon. As Dr. Robert Austrian has demonstrated, the disease is still there, but we no longer recognize it and usually get rid of it in its earliest stages. Most of today's young physicians have never seen a case of diphtheria or meningococcal meningitis or erysipelas. Even tuberculosis, which used to require whole, immense hospitals because of the enormous numbers of tuberculous patients, has almost disappeared. Syphilis is still around, to be sure, but chiefly in the early, acute stages of the disease. Because of peni-cillin, tertiary syphilis, which was among the commonest causes of heart disease, paralysis, and insanity just a few decades ago, has virtually gone out of medicine.

The clinical research that made all this possible was accomplished mainly during the 1940s and 1950s. During this time, institutions like the Thorndike Memorial Laboratories of the Boston City Hospital devoted a large part of their resources to the testing and evaluation of new and improved antibiotics. The knowledge about these substances as antibacterial substances and their mode of action against various bacteria came, by and large, from the research ventures of skilled microbiological laboratories. But the knowledge of these substances as medicines for use in the treatment of disease in human beings had to come from careful, meticulous, scrupulously scientific clinical research. This was, if you will, human experimentation.

I suggest that this experience in clinical investigation spanning more than two decades in teaching hospital centers here and abroad was the largest-scale undertaking in human experimentation that the world has known. I suggest, therefore, that if you want to find out more about how this kind of research is best done, as well as where its weaknesses are, there is no better model to examine than this one. Everything else that medicine has accomplished thus far in the line of scientific research involving human subjects has been relatively minor both in sheer scale as well as in significance for human welfare. If there are basic flaws in the whole concept of human experimentation, you ought to be able to demonstrate these flaws in the long history of antibiotic research. And if you wish to introduce reforms into the existing system for research of this kind in order to assure against inequities and injustice in the future, you should be careful to keep the record of antibiotic research in mind as you go. For a starter in this line of inquiry, I would suggest a careful study of the voluminous and illuminating bibliography of Dr. Maxwell Finland, whose work on antibiotics and antibacterial chemotherapy covers the whole period from 1937 up to the present decade.

I do not raise this matter because I wish to indicate unqualified support for the idea of human experimentation or even to suggest that the work on antibiotics was done flawlessly. Certainly, here and there, the record displays experiments that should not have been done or in which the patient's welfare was not the central concern, although I doubt the existence of any such examples in Dr. Finland's bibliography. I raise it because of a concern that it may be overlooked in today's vigorous and sometimes violent arguments over issues of human experimentation in which the stakes are very much lower and even, on occasion, trivial. I would hate to see us lay down restrictions or sanctions on clinical science in general on the basis of today's apprehensions about psychosurgery or behavior control or sex determination or genetic engineering and the like. I would hope that each of these would be considered as isolated problems, on their own merits or demerits, without any implications whatever for the general question as to whether or not human experimentation should be done. It worries me that there is so much public attention being drawn to what seem to me quite esoteric zones of science, while the *real* agenda, the major problems in human disease still unsolved, stares us full in the face.

The truth is that we have a very long way to go in medicine. It is simply not true that medical science has progressed so rapidly and marvelously that our main concern should now be how to cope with the technology that has replaced the art. Except for a handful of conspicuous advances, such as the antibiotics, several vitamins, and a number of hormones, we are still confronted by enormous areas of ignorance about disease, and we would do well to acknowledge these more often than we publicly do. Let me just mention a few to convey an idea of the scope of ignorance.

We do not understand the underlying mechanisms of heart disease at all. There are clues to suggest the basis for arteriosclerosis and valvular disease, but nothing yet with the stature of solid scientific proof. We must therefore remain without effective measures either for the prevention or the cure of heart disease.

We do not yet have an understanding of the pathogenesis of cancer, and because of this lack we have no immediate prospects of either reversing or preventing the process of neoplasia. We cannot explain the mechanisms involved in stroke. We know how to lower the blood pressure in hypertension, but it is still no certainty that we have learned how to prevent the vascular lesions of this disorder. We can neither prevent nor reverse the pathological processes in chronic glomerulonephritis or pyelonephritis, the chief causes of renal failure, and there is therefore nothing to offer beyond dialysis or transplantation in these diseases. We do not really understand bronchial asthma or chronic pulmonary fibrosis or hepatic cirrhosis or multiple sclerosis or senile dementia or schizophrenia or rheumatoid arthritis or the vascular disease that kills people with diabetes despite insulin or peptic ulcer or even migraine.

I could go on with the dismal litany, although not forever, for it is a finite list amounting to some twenty-five or thirty major diseases that account for most of the premature deaths and incapacitations among us. These are the diseases that fill the modern hospitals, and the lack of knowledge concerning their mechanisms accounts for the absence of effective technologies to prevent or cure them. This general lack, in turn, accounts in greatest part for the enormous cost of health care in our society. As it happens all of these diseases are now recognized as respectable, approachable, and potentially soluble biological problems.

Personally, I have not the slightest doubt that we will obtain clear answers, sooner or later, for all of them, with the same certainty that now allows us to deal effectively with the major part of human infectious disease. But the answers and the final technologies will not drop into our laps, nor will we arrive at them by guesswork or by good luck. What we must have, if we wish to become a reasonably healthy species, is a great deal of new information. Much of this will only be obtainable by clinical science; that is to say, by experimentation involving human disease. This has to be faced up to as we deliberate here about the necessary guidelines for the medical research of the future.

THE RISKS OF RESEARCH

Walsh McDermott

As Dr. Thomas has so eloquently described it, he and I date from the days of iron men and wooden ships in which I had a slight advantage over him, in that my year as an intern was the last one without sulfonamide. So, I had the opportunity to see, as a physician, the introduction of this era that he has described.

I also share with him completely the idea that the clinical investigation in the field of microbial diseases presented virtually all of the problems with which we are faced today. There are, however, a few important differences, as there always are, in the use of models, and I shall attempt to highlight those as I go along.

I would like to add one footnote to what he was saying. In the clinical investigation of microbial diseases there were times when the total supply of the new, powerful, and for the first time effective drug was in very small supply and was needed for certain purposes, social purposes, if you will. The entire supply of penicillin had to be controlled for the use of the military because we were in the middle of World War II. This was done through the National Academy of Sciences-National Research Council mechanism. It was done, in effect, within this building. But the ethical questions as to who got what had to be determined by military considerations. Consequently, when it was demonstrated that penicillin was of very great effectiveness in treating syphilis, its uses for that purpose became an investigative question of great moment.

It was also demonstrated at that same time that penicillin was highly effective in subacute bacterial endocarditis, an essentially uniformly fatal disease, but one of no interest to the military. So we had then an essentially nonfatal disease in which penicillin could be given and a fatal disease in which it could not. Two men were dominating the scene as the respective chairmen of the committees within this house, one the late Dr. Chester Keefer and the other Dr. Joseph Earl Moore. I was present in Dr. Moore's office when a woman called up and stated that she had just talked to Dr. Keefer and had told him that if her husband could not receive penicillin for his bacterial endocarditis, she was going to send him out to get syphilis so that he could get the drug from Dr. Moore.

Dr. Thomas, of course, has told us of one kind of risk of research, namely, that the research does not get done. I interpret my assignment to talk about the risks to the participant subject in the research. By *risk* I mean that someone is placed at a risk of dangers that would not have happened had that person not been a participant in the research. By *experiment* I mean either on the first occasion of new observational techniques within the human body or the choosing of some intervention in the course of human disease or human condition and subjecting that intervention to experiment.

Every medical intervention has some risk; and, as Dr. Francis Moore states, every medical procedure is in itself an experiment. But there is a difference here; specifically, the difference of experience. The surgical procedure that has been done before is different than that surgical procedure that has never been done. The drug that has been received by fifty people is a slightly different proposition than the drug that has never been received by anyone, and so it goes.

There then is a quantitative aspect to experience. The more experience, the less a particular intervention could be considered an experiment; the less experience, the more. It is a rather arbitrary point at times, yet one that can be reasonably well settled. But the nature of the risks run a spectrum all the way from a petty annoyance -- hives, let us say, or some such thing -- to death. That is, any type of a reaction that can occur to any type of medical intervention represents a danger that can be present and through which a participant in research can be put at risk. It is impossible, therefore, really, to have risk-free participation in a research project.

The risks can come from any quarter. A new drug for hypertension can turn out to be a better drug than the existing treatment, in which case the people who got the new drug were at less risk than the people who got the old. Or it could turn out not so well. Therefore, they were put at greater risk. The subjects on the drug would be put at greater risk of toxicity, for the toxicity is not yet known; or it could turn out that the risks were actually less. So there are any number of ways that risk occurs here. But everyone participating in the question gets put at some risk or another.

Now, obviously there can be a whole set of issues that arise as a result of this question of risks. There is the question of the nature of the risks. There is the question of their reduction or amelioration. There is the question of how much the participant should know. There are the societal trade-offs between the risks to the individual and to society -- risks to the individual as someone with a particular disease, a person in a particular case; the risk to an individual simply as a member of society; and the risk to society. And then, by what right does one human being place another at risk? These are some of the issues that come to mind when considering the risks of research. As I mentioned, any participation can give any type of reaction to a medical intervention. But generally speaking, the risks are of four main kinds.

The first has to do with direct trauma from physical damage by some new observational technique or by a severe tissue reaction to some substance that has been injected. The second is damage to an organ or organ system as a result of drug toxicity. The third is the withholding of a treatment of established value. But the fourth is the question of the risks coming from the associated tests set up to test the risks and to protect against them. This is a sleeper in the risk business in clinical investigation, and one on which I will elaborate in a moment.

The first two require little comment, for there are various ways of guarding against drug toxicity or minimizing it, and this is also true of observational technique. The question of the tests is that various diagnostic tests in medicine all have trade-offs between the risk of the test and the risk of the condition for which the test is being designed. Sometimes the test itself carries with it a considerable degree of danger, but it is aimed at and helps in the identification of something very serious and of very great importance to the patient.

A contemporary example does not come to mind at the moment, but a relatively recent one does, namely, aspiration of sternal marrow. Although this procedure is no longer very much in use, it is an extremely useful one in establishing certain forms of disease of the blood-forming organs. Among all the areas new drugs are most apt to affect are the blood-forming organs. Accordingly, when one is setting up a clinical investigation of a new drug and attempting to protect the patient against any ills that might befall him, one watches the blood-forming organ system very carefully. The question in writing the protocol then arises as to whether or not to do sternal marrows. The procedure itself has acquired a familiarity in hospital service. There are a lot of blood disease procedures done all the time, done perfectly as far as trade-offs are concerned, and so this procedure has acquired a sanctity that has only to do with its use as a diagnostic procedure in a patient who may have a hematologic disease. Having acquired that sanctity, when someone asks if sternal marrows are to be done, you say, "Sure." So, the first thing you know, the patient who is actually at risk only of a theoretical damage to the blood-forming organs is receiving an observational method aimed at protecting him but actually increasing the risk. I emphasize that this particular example is not one that is current. But this is the sort of thing that comes in waves as tests come in and out, and I am sure will appear again. Therefore, one of the sleepers in risks in clinical investigation is to be sure that the very tests you are applying to protect the patient are not themselves adding considerably to the risk.

The last of the four kinds of risk is withholding, and this is really the area of greatest problems. In starkest terms it has to do with withholding the intervention from one group of people and making the intervention in the other, a so-called "control group." This gets us into the question of random selection in clinical trials, which I would like to discuss in a moment.

Withholding today is rarely so simple as some individuals getting drug A while others get nothing. Usually it has to do with the decision to withhold drug A while introducing drug B, a new drug for the same purpose. This dates back, of course, to those days that Dr. Thomas mentioned when one could give sulfonamide to a patient secure in the knowledge that all that medical science could do was being done. But the minute another drug was introduced, the question arose, is it fair to the patient to try to study penicillin in pneumococcal pneumonia without at the same time giving him sulfonamide? If one gave both drugs, it was impossible to determine the effectiveness of the new one; but if both drugs were not given, one was making an ethical decision specifically putting the patient at risk of the possible dangers of not receiving the known drug. So the withholding issue gets to be right away a very difficult one from an ethical standpoint once there are multiple drugs available.

A big step occurs at that very point. I have been talking here of results of a single investigation, a single team, a single investigator with associates on a single service. The withholding phenomenon comes to even greater importance today in the question of the large-scale cooperative study aimed at defining the validity of some intervention.

For two decades or more the tool of the large-scale cooperative study with random selection of the experimental subjects has been fashionable. This system, as you know, is based on the premise that one can identify a large group of people all having the same disease and having it in the same stages, the same subsets, so that the behavior of that disease can be predictable in such a large group. Then by some process of random selection, one assigns to some groups the intervention, and to other groups nothing at all or another form of intervention. The introduction of this random-selection, large-scale study represented a laudable attempt for introducing rigor into this very difficult question of the validation of various procedures.

Now, I have long contended that insofar as therapies are concerned -- I am not now talking about vaccines -- by the time the ethical questions are met in such a large-scale study, the tool is really of relatively little value. By this time you are reduced to studying questions that no one is very deeply concerned about, that people have more or less made up their own minds about, and that cannot be classified as burning, acute questions.

So, this is an elaborate, tedious, hard-working process that by the time all the wheels turn, in my judgment, is only usable in a set of questions that are valuable enough but not major. The reason that I do not consider it a valuable procedure is that, because the assignment of participants to various groups is decided by chance, no one can really be asked to take very excessive risks. In effect, an experiment has been set up in which there is something for everybody, and all of the participants tend to get some form of accepted intervention. The experiment itself then comes down to comparing which intervention is superior. Although this is useful for discarding therapies, it seldom is capable of answering critical questions.

One cannot generalize on the morality of the random selection because every case is different. These are things about which honest men can differ, and a great deal depends on the nature of the intervention that is under study and the nature of the research project.

How can these four categories of risk be avoided or minimized? I won't dwell on the drug toxicity other than to say that from the anti-microbial drug days I can tell of serious reactions that were drug dependent and that would not have occurred had we known proper dosage. I can think of at least two, the vestibular dysfunction of streptomycin and the anemia of chloramphenicol, serious reactions that occurred in considerable numbers in humans and that were subsequently shown to be producible in dogs. But there are ways of minimizing drug toxicity, and they are pretty well standardized. In addition we must maintain a continuous awareness, a continuous scrutiny of the protective tests mentioned earlier, and above all a climate of openness. Special research services, with signs over the door, are helpful. This is, of course, not economically possible everywhere, but I believe it is definitely helpful, because it preserves this climate of openness that is really the only essential thing we have.

One should remember such points as that an antimicrobial drug with toxicity that is quite acceptable as a therapeutic agent may be quite unacceptable as a chemoprophylactic agent. In the one instance you are treating people by the hundreds who are quite seriously ill. In the other instance, you are treating people by the thousands and hundreds of thousands, none of whom is ill when you start. The differences there can be quite important. But above all, we must persist in maintaining the climate of openness and a careful challenge of the importance and the validity of the research questions. One must be sure that the game really is worth the candle, and that one has a perfect experiment rather than an imperfect experiment.

There are times, however, when a less than perfect experiment produces a less than definitive answer, but a building block emerges on which something else can be done. For example, during the Korean War, it was shown that whole blood was essential for battlefield casualties. The whole blood was, of course, contaminated with hepatitis virus, and a number of different attempts were being made to inactivate the virus. These had to be studied experimentally in human subjects, there being no other model that showed it. The work, as I recall, was done in human volunteers who would receive the blood containing the known virus, which was then inactivated in various ways. The question of design was whether it was necessary in each instance, in addition to giving the subject the virus laden blood plus the inactivator, to give blood without any inactivator in order to show that the virus was still present. Those would be the conditions of a perfect experiment. In an imperfect experiment one would simply be satisfied with giving the blood and the inactivator, and then, if it were shown enough times that that procedure resulted in a reduced incidence of the disorder, to work the thing up more classically.

Other things have to do with withholdings there, and Dr. Moore's point about the biology of disease is tremendously important. We get bemused by the expression "outcome results" and forget that sometimes we do know a little bit of what is going on. Sometimes in studies of patients treated, comparing, for example, the hospital with the home, the issue in outcome results is not the benefits of home cooking, but rather if there is some particular intervention that is being done in the hospital that cannot be delivered to the home in any circumstance.

For example, when it was thought that hospital treatment was absolutely essential for the proper treatment of tuberculosis, chemotherapy came on the scene. It then was clear that the critical element in the treatment of tuberculosis was the introduction of a chemical into the human body, a chemical that would interfere with the metabolic processes of the tubercle bacillus. This was something that could be delivered both at hospital and at home. A study was done to prove it and did so quite well. But there are other diseases in which what is available in a hospital, such as some highly technical machinery, is not available in the home. One could study a considerable group of patients both at hospital and home without seeing any difference in outcome, provided the need for use of the complicated machinery was something that arose only very rarely. So one has to challenge each large-scale clinical test on the withholding issue to be sure that all of the patients are protected against whatever it is that is being studied and that nothing is being withheld that could lead to serious disease or death. In our preoccupation with outcome, we tend to forget that the two groups can have the same outcome; but one or two individuals within the group could have a very sad outcome, indeed, and one that was preventable.

In closing I will reiterate my position, namely, that it is impossible to do clinical investigation without putting people at some risk. In many instances the risk is an unknown one, and in many instances the risk can be cut down. Nevertheless, it is impossible to do investigations without putting some people at some risk.

Who is to make the decisions on those risks? I have written my position on this elsewhere, and I will simply state it briefly here. In the first place, much can be taken care of simply by interchange between the investigator and the subject. I quite agree that informed consent is something that is grossly manipulatable. But as long as there is a reasonable understanding back and forth on many of these questions, the degree of risk is not such that it is asking too much for the patient to assume, presuming they know what they are doing. However, there come times when the decision is much more than that.

Whenever in our society we make a decision that could harm an individual, we try to institutionalize it. We set up draft boards. We have judicial procedures. We have trial by jury. My position is that we have not yet arrived at that point in our society in regard to the use of human subjects in experimentation and research. Nor is there, so far as I can see, any foreseeable way in which we can. The various mechanisms we do have, the human experimentation committees and all the rest, I think are fine. They serve to maintain this climate of openness and these challenges for the investigator. But we have not institution-alized any way in which we can say that it is proper for an investigator to go ahead and study a given question. Yet, there are times when it simply has to be done and that an investigator will put other people at risk. However much one may surround those times with climates of open-ness and with challenges, and I think this should be the case, however much one may quite properly invoke the trust that is the wonderful thing between the physician and his patient in its finest moments, there is no one who can relieve the investigator from assuming that responsibil-ity and making the decision to put another person at risk.

INQUIRY AND COMMENTARY

FREDERICK ROBBINS: Our three speakers are now available to you to answer questions, to clarify, and they also are quite free to communicate among themselves in regard to some of the issues that they have discussed.

I would like to take the prerogative of asking the first question by requesting Dr. McDermott to elaborate a bit further on clinical trials. I would like him to comment on the value of establishing the validity of something by clinical trial in a cost effective sort of a way, as opposed to not establishing its validity. Let us take tonsil and adenoidectomy as an example. This has, to my knowledge, never been subjected to a true clinical trial. Would you estimate what the cost of that might have been?

McDERMOTT: You are dealing with the illusion of a rational world. If that particular procedure had been validated by clinical trial, in-numerable lives would have been saved. Psychiatrists can tell us all the wonderful nonconsequences from the early childhood trauma of the procedure, and so forth, yet no clinical trial was done. But the procedure is now discarded. That is, the conventional wisdom, at long last, has gotten rid of it.

ROBBINS: Can you document that statement?

McDERMOTT: I think you can if you look through the textbooks, different editions of textbooks. If you look at pediatrics textbooks --

ROBBINS: I am not talking about textbooks. I am asking about what goes on in hospitals.

McDERMOTT: Well, let me answer the question this way. You asked me to elaborate on clinical trials. Specifically, you cannot subject a procedure to random selection at the moment of its inception. The moment somebody gets an idea about tonsillectomy, or the moment somebody introduces a new drug, one cannot, at that point, subject the procedure to random selection and clinical trial. One has to get some information about it and some feel for it before there is enough experience to put it out on a clinical trial.

Now, in the very process of obtaining that information, the people who are doing it get some feel for the validity of the procedure, they get a conviction. They believe that what they are doing is effective, and this belief spreads to other physicians. So by the time you are ready for the clinical trial, and if what you are experimenting with is a very powerful and effective agent for some very serious risk, physicians are not willing to put to a random process the choice as to whether their patient does or does not get this intervention, because by now they have come to believe in it. Therefore, you can only put out to clinical trials those questions about which large blocks of the profession have pretty well made up their minds or rather unimportant questions about which people have not made up their minds.

The tonsillectomy is a splendid example of the type of intervention that gets into our armamentarium and stays there against most people's belief in its validity. The textbooks certainly state that it is not valid. If you think that doing a clinical trial would take it out of business, well and good. It would certainly be stopped when doctors are no longer reimbursed for the procedure by health insurance or Social Security.

HOWARD HIATT: I am Dean of the Harvard School of Public Health. I would like to address a question to Dr. Moore. He expressed concern for increasing federal intervention in the process of medical care. I think that it is a concern that all of us who have been involved in patient care and human experimentation share. On the other hand, an aroused American public and Congress many years ago felt constrained to pass a set of laws that created a Food and Drug Administration to regulate the use of drugs. I wonder what suggestions Dr. Moore might offer with respect to similar controls for the use of medical procedures and surgical procedures, such as tonsillectomy. Despite a general consensus on the part of physicians, as you have just expressed, Dr. McDermott, and I think Dr. Robbins, agrees, a million tonsillectomies were carried out in the United States last year. Dr. Moore can cite many more than I can, innumerable procedures that have come into the culture that have been carried out in large numbers only to have been abandoned. Everybody comments about the procedure called "gastric freezing" for ulcer disease that became popular in the early 1960s, and it finally disappeared. It disappeared not because a better procedure has come along for the treatment of ulcer disease -- that would have been quite appropriate -- but because it has been shown to be without merit. But that occurred only after several thousands of people had been subjected to the

44

procedure at a considerable economic cost and an even greater human cost. You can cite large numbers of procedures that can be described in similar terms. At the present time we know that sweeping the country is the coronary artery bypass graft procedure for coronary artery disease, and while that may have a place --

ROBBINS: Dr. Sabin and I don't want to examine that too carefully, since we are both recipients.

HIATT: You have anticipated my saying that while there are defenders, and defenders for good reason of the procedure in some patients, it certainly has not extended beyond the area in which it could be called an experiment. And yet its price has yet to be established in precise ways. We are not doing what might be termed a pilot experiment. We are doing this procedure on literally tens of thousands of people -- again at enormous economic and human cost -- and we have no regulatory procedure that permits us to place this operation in its rightful role before it then becomes as widespread as it should be or as it should not be.

Dr. Moore, I share your view that we want as little in the way of intervention as is necessary that might interfere with the relationship of the physician and his or her patient in the proper advance of medical knowledge. But surely unless some kind of regulation is introduced, we are going to find it introduced from the outside. Clearly the membership of this meeting denotes the fact that medicine no longer belongs to the physician alone. It is the area that belongs to all of science. What mechanisms can the physician, the clinical investigator, the professor of surgery, the professor of medicine, society in general take that will correct some of these inequities without introducing the unwarranted interference that you, so rightfully, are concerned about?

MOORE: In the first place, I did not say that I was opposed to federal intervention in any aspect of medicine, although generally I think it should be examined closely. What I said was that these difficult problems of the ethical aspects of experimental work in people cannot be settled by some sort of federal fiat. They could not be settled by state fiat or county fiat or city fiat or village fiat. You cannot do this sort of thing by governmental edict. We have to rely on the development of an open society, on institutions that know how to do these things rightfully and safely. The federal area already is deeply in this field through a limitation on funding of NIH grants unless certain human-use procedures are gone through. I liked Dr. McDermott's statement that is pretty much all right the way it is, that it challenges the investigator to say what he is doing, and it favors openness. Openness and young people are the two great saviors we have. So I would answer Dr. Hiatt's question by saying that I don't think that the federal government should try to settle something like this with a single rule or law. You just cannot do it.

Now I would like to backtrack a little bit. It always interests me the way physicians bring up surgical operations. So I will take the liberty of asking about the use of the new oral hypoglycemic agents, which are widely used without really much knowledge of how they do. How about the potent new digitalis drugs? How about propanolol? This using of new things on people is not wholly confined to surgical operations; they are part of the whole fabric of medicine. A forum like this is an appropriate place to bring out this point. And again I would challenge Dr. Hiatt. He really is believing in the illusion of a rational society if he believes that all the soft and difficult areas in that huge field can be controlled by governmental fiat.

Finally, I would like to comment about tonsillectomy. We have just finished a massive study of surgery in this country, and tonsillectomy is still done in huge numbers. My own feeling is that it is unnecessary and unwise. But we are going to see it disappear, just the way radiation of little babies for so-called "enlargement of the thymus" disappeared. And it is going to disappear by the ripple effect. Dr. Robbins has challenged us to show by hospital records that tonsillectomy is on the wane. He will find the answer if he will look at his own major teaching hospital ENT service as we looked at the Massachusetts Eye and Ear Infirmary. There we found that they are doing about 5 percent of what they used to; and when those residents get out, I think we will see the disappearance of this blight.

It is also interesting in regard to coronary artery bypass surgery -- and I recommend to all of you the recent readings sponsored by Dr. Ingelfinger in the *New England Journal of Medicine* -- that in order to do a controlled clinical trial on that procedure we really have got to bite an awfully hard bullet, because you would have to do an open thoracotomy and dissectomy before you really knew where you were with it, and that is going to be rough stuff.

JOAN GOLDSTEIN: I am the National Coordinator for the Women's Health Task Force for the National Organization for Women. My question is for Dr. Moore.

You gave as illustrations of persons who volunteered happily for medical experimentation those who were critically or seriously ill, those for whom there was no hope. You did not include or mention in that group persons who were not ill but who by other sources are drawn in as subjects in medical experimentation. I think there is a need to add to that list persons whom it is decided are eligible to be medically experimented upon.

Then there was your illustration from the Warsaw Ghetto of the physicians who documented the starvation experience of their fellow sufferers. I believe you were making a mild point when you said that if the victim documents the victimization then it is a morally acceptable point of view; that is, if it were Jewish doctors who were documenting Jewish starvation then it is a morally acceptable point. I think what you are raising in my mind, anyway, is that the concept

46

of informed consent is not clearly defined or has not been defined
clearly enough so that we can deal with the issue at this Forum. I
would hope that it would be the point of this conference to have a
clear definition of the concept of informed consent and its ability
to be applied and also monitored. Therefore, I am asking you,
Dr. Moore, what do you instruct persons working with you in surgery
or as surgeons of what is informed consent? How do you teach that
concept? How do you define it, and how is it applied?

MOORE: I think you have three things in there that I will try to dissect
out. One of them had to do with persons that were not subject to
experiment but were also involved with it. I am not really sure I
know what you mean. But since you speak especially from the women's
point of view, I will bring out the fact that we currently have in
the world today the most gigantic human experimentation ever undertaken: the wide dissemination of oral contraceptive medication, which
is not yet well understood and which is being used on a vast scale.
The people who are taking those pills are women. So that is something we should bear in mind.

Secondly, as to informed consent, it is a contradiction in terms
because it is an experiment into the unknown. No one can inform
you as to the results. There is another position, and that is that
the person involved should have the very areas of uncertainty and
ignorance explained to him or her. This, of course, should be done.
In answer to the recent question, this is what we tried to do, and
I think I was merely trying to call attention to the fact that the
term *informed consent* is a kind of a trap. What we really mean is
full explanation and a normal, relaxed human exchange between the
so-called expert and the so-called subject.

ALBERT SABIN: I have set down three points in Dr. Moore's very admirable
address. Two of them have already been raised. First of all, I will
address myself to the interpretation of fact, and I would not have
raised this point about the ultimate significance of experiments
with human fetal tissue in the development of the polio vaccination
if the same point he made were not made in precisely the same way in
an editorial this morning in the *Washington Post* and if I had not
been receiving innumerable letters.

When Dr. Enders referred to this in his Nobel address, he indicated that about forty years ago I had done such experiments, and
then some years later they did something in the laboratory there.
I would like to say that I wish I had never done that experiment.
It was an absolute blind alley. I used the wrong strain, which made
it impossible to progress and actually was a blockade to knowledge.
I think the ultimate development of polio vaccine rested on other
things, and especially the admirable development of the new tissue
culture techniques by Enders and Weller and Robbins, about which
there is no argument.

But I do wish to still say something about federal regulations, even though this has already been discussed very fully by Dr. Hiatt. Dr. Moore has a wonderful way of resolving things, and perhaps he will resolve a little more his statement that it is not always necessary to solve problems by federal regulations. I find the key word here to be *always*. But then he went on to say that laws cannot entirely protect against evil people. That is also true, but we must ask what is the alternative? Is it no laws at all, or is it the best laws we can devise? And therefore, I would ask Dr. Moore to indicate whether or not the issue really is federal regulation or no federal regulation -- and let us substitute *national* for *federal*, which is already a kind of dirty word -- and further ask him whether it is not an issue of what kind of national regulation is prudent and what is not prudent? Ultimately we have to get down to concrete facts, and I would like to hear Dr. Moore comment on that.

ROBBINS: I would like to simply comment on your factual statement, which I disagree with to some extent. But I would discuss this with you at a later time, because Dr. Moore is going to have to leave.

SABIN: On that one thing I don't want to be misunderstood. I could make up a list of things that are needed for progress -- and fetal tissues are of absolute importance for further progress -- but I would like to base it on a more reliable foundation than the one like the polio vaccine.

MOORE: I think that for me to discuss the use of fetal tissue in the presence of Dr. Sabin and Dr. Robbins would be the height of ridiculousness. I would only say, Dr. Robbins, that you cannot get out of it that easily. I think Dr. Sabin has just said the thing that needed to be said: that is, while one may have a variation in interpretation as to the particularly critical nature of the use of human fetal tissue and the history of Dr. Enders' work, nonetheless, the importance of being able to use it for certain things, of course, is unquestioned.

Now, to go on to the other point. I agree with Dr. Sabin's modification that some sort of national guidelines or national statement or national push towards challenge and openness is appropriate. The only thing I am trying to avoid, again, is what I perceive of as an American tendency to identify a problem and then to become overspecific and overregulatory with it, putting the society in a very difficult situation. Dr. McDermott put it very well in saying that this is a very complicated problem and not one that is readily given to simplistic federal solutions. Do you want to comment some more on that?

McDERMOTT: I would like to say just one thing, namely, we have been talking in terms of legislative enactments or administrative agency decisions. There are other aspects of society's laws here, and one

48

of them is the concept of due care in case law. We have distinguished members of the bar in the audience who know far more about this than I do. But I simply point this out as one other mechanism that society has to establish some of the safeguards that Dr. Thomas was talking about in the beginning -- safeguards, I think, that every person who looks at the situation believes we should have.

SAMUEL GOROVITZ: I am Professor and Chairman of the Department of Philosophy at the University of Maryland. It seems to me that there are two assumptions that have pervaded the discussion thus far. Both of them I find quite congenial. The first is that medical research has some very good consequences, and the second is that federal regulation potentially threatens to constrain medical research in a most unwelcome way.

I think both of those points are true and important. I enjoyed very much Dr. Moore's historical remarks. It does seem to me, however, that they are primarily a history of the benefits and successes of experimentation in medicine rather than a history of experimentation in medicine. I think we are all aware that there have been rather serious abuses of the privilege of experimentation, and those abuses have involved the imposition of a variety of risks on the subjects of those experimentations. Dr. McDermott gave us what I view as an important but incomplete cataloging of those risks. It seems to me there are many kinds of risks that his catalog excludes. I would like to step back for a minute and ask why a forum like this is taking place?

I think the reason that it is timely and important for an event such as this to take place is that the view of the risks and benefits of medical research that has currency within medical practice and medical research -- and, I should say, even the spectrum of views that have currency within medical practice and medical research -- stand quite apart from certain kinds of views that have currency outside the medical world. There are people who view medical research as predominantly unsavory and not as predominantly beneficial.

There are people who view the risks as having a magnitude that in general overrides what they see as the benefits. I think some of those critics of the research establishment have a nostalgia for a past that never existed, and they would be much benefited by hearing some of the history of the successes of medical research. But they focus on a different aspect of that history, that is, the abuses and in some instances the egregious and indefensible abuses. They see federal regulation in a detailed and comprehensive form as necessary to protect against risks of the four kinds that we have been told about and risks of other kinds as well, not just risks of physical injury but risks of psychological damage, of the overriding of personal autonomy, of being victimized by unethical practices even in the absence of physical damage.

I believe it is important for the scientific community, if it is effectively to succeed in its attempt to retain the privilege of being the primary source of its own control and regulation, to exhibit clearly a sensitivity to and understanding of the motivations that prompt the press for external regulations. If we are to successfully constrain the increase of federal controls, I think we have to exhibit a better understanding of its origins, or at least of the origins of the motivation that gives rise to it. That motivation arises out of a broader perception of the risks that are at issue.

I wonder then if we could not to some extent broaden the context of our inquiry by focusing a bit more explicity some attention on what happens on the darker side of the history of experimentation and by looking somewhat more explicity not at the glories, which I take it we all are willing to acknowledge, but at the horrors. In this way we might come to an understanding of why it is that widely abroad in the land there is public concern that people involved in medical and clinical research ought not to be allowed to continue to do what they have done in the past.

I address these remarks to anyone who cares to respond.

LEWIS THOMAS: I am not sure what some examples of this darker side would be. How general are they? How widely can we extrapolate from them? Is it the habit of clinical research in this country to be living on this dark and unperceived side, or are these exceptional? Could you give us a few examples of what you have in mind?

GOROVITZ: I think there is one mistake in the response that you have just made in your question, and that is the suggestion that it is critically important how widespread these darker, unperceived sides of research are. The point I am trying to make is precisely that it is perceived more broadly than its occurrence would warrant. All you need is one Willowbrook, one Tuskegee, one instance of dramatic front-page stuff, and you have a ground swell of reaction across the nation. One report on research with fetal heads, and this is what to the body politic medical research is about.

Now, it may be that the horror stories constitute what, from the inside, is a statistically insignificant percentage of medical research. It is precisely that point, it seems to me, that leads to a distorted perception on the part of medical researchers of what the problem is. The problem is that the perspective that the public has of medical research is not a perspective from the inside. It is not a perspective that perceives the occasional abuse in the context of a broad pattern of success undertaken in the context of integrity. Rather the public view, to an increasing extent, I believe, is to extrapolate from the abuses and to characterize the whole thereby. The proper address to that, it seems to me, cannot be simply to say, "Those abuses are too insignificant for us to take seriously," because it just won't wash.

MOORE: I would just like to say that I absolutely agree with
Mr. Gorovitz. I think that we do have a tendency to look at the
good side of this. In my little talk I mentioned briefly the
Krebiozen business as being a very dark chapter. But I think the
most important message he has given us is one that we can apply to
many things. We have to understand how other people perceive us,
whenever we are speaking of medicine and medical research, in order
to understand how we can help assist in understanding and communication. One of the things that we have tried to do is to analyze the
functional anatomy of successful, or what we might perceive of as
ethically acceptable human experimentation. It might be quite worthwhile to gather together some of these very sad chapters that
Mr. Gorovitz has mentioned and then try to dissect the anatomy of
those particular episodes to see what happened, to see some of these
things having to do with the man, the institution, the question of
openness, ego drive, and scientific rivalry. If we would begin to
see them on the other side, I think that would be an interesting
exercise to undertake.

McDERMOTT: I see no way out of this. Once it had been shown that research with human subjects produced information of use for mankind
in general -- for example, once it was possible to drive yellow fever
out of the cities of the Americas and build the Panama Canal -- it
was clear that society has a stake in doing such research.
   The dark side, as far as I can see -- and I think I probably know
many chapters in it -- is one human being putting another human being
at risk. Although my contention is that you cannot do one without
the other, you can do a lot to help, to ameliorate. You can challenge people to ask if a question or an experiment is really necessary. But having done that, there remain times when somebody simply
has to put somebody at risk if the societal rights, if you will, are
to have the results of useful research that will come through. Now,
I don't see any way to institutionalize that type of problem. I
regard it as a great moral dilemma.

ALBERT MORACZEWSKI: I am from the Pope John XXIII Medical Moral Research
and Education Center in St. Louis, Missouri. I was glad that
Dr. Moore had the opportunity to expand his remark about informed
consent, because I was concerned about his earlier interpretation.
   I would like to focus specifically on this: What precisely is
the relationship between the experimenter and the experimentee or
the physician and the subject? How does the physician view this
relationship? Does he see it as one of parent to child, teacher to
student, master to disciple, or as one of partners in a cooperative
venture? I think this attitude, the one that each investigator must
clarify for himself, will determine the way he approaches informed
consent. When there are large numbers of subjects there is the
danger of passing them routinely and of forgetting the human dignity
of each subject, regardless of his intelligence, his background, his

class, age, or his condition. If the investigator approaches each individual subject as a coinvestigator in a project, then I feel some of the abuses may be reduced because the basic correct attitude of respect for the other would be present. I would then ask the panel if they wish to agree or disagree, or if they would accept this idea of seeing the subject as coexperimenter.

ROBBINS: Are there comments from the panel? I think we find this an acceptable point of view.

MOORE: I think it is a very acceptable point of view, and you will see many articles in the literature in which the subjects are coauthors. The spiritual point you have made is a very, very important one. There are times when communications are difficult, and it is not always possible to enlist large numbers of cohorts into such a relationship. But if an investigator has that degree of human respect for the relationship, it certainly helps.

H. HUGH FUDENBERG: I would like to make one comment and ask a question. Dr. Gorovitz raised the question to which the panel responded in part. I gather he was suggesting that in order for biomedical research to proceed with minimal delay that it would be adequate to require really informed consent not only of subjects but also of the American public. I think both scientists and science writers have been remiss in not educating the American public as to how biomedical research is performed and in highlighting only those few abuses with which we are all familiar. In case any of you are interested, there is a new organization called the Biological Alliance that is dedicated to writing articles on how such work is done for one hundred newspapers throughout the country. One reason we are here is to interview the big ones personally. But the thing of such proportions for those of you who are not physicians has other aspects. In most university hospitals it is not possible to take excess urine that is discarded after urinalysis or the excess few drops of blood discarded after blood is drawn for a blood test and use them to work out some new tests that could then be standardized for a new diagnosis of disease without getting the written consent of the person involved. I think this is perhaps being carried to illogical extremes of informed consent. Perhaps educating the American public will be of help.

Now, my specific question is addressed to both Dr. Thomas and Dr. McDermott. You have indicated that there are two kinds of risks essentially that the patient runs, sins of commission and sins of omission. For the sins of omission, you mentioned not giving, for example, sulfonamide and giving penicillin instead. Nowadays we need informed consent for that.

Let us take the example of the choice of a physician not to do a tonsillectomy under conditions when the textbook calls for it or not to radiate the thymus of an infant when the thymus was enlarged.

I would think that that type of "sin" of omission could be incurred at times and very well disregarded by the entire medical community and the entire populace unless a lawsuit might arise from such a sin of omission by someone who was ill-informed. I am sure that new examples of this will arise in the next several years. Standard procedures will be discarded by someone without getting a human experimentation consent form. My question to you, Dr. McDermott, is how would you answer that?

My question to Dr. Thomas specifically is: Do you think that taking out the tonsils and adenoids in view of the recent literature might create cancer some twenty or twenty-five years down the road. If so, how do we keep records of things that might have very late masses of patients if they are done and are accepted procedures?

McDERMOTT: As to the first man to challenge the conventional wisdom of a procedure, I think that represents one of the reasons why it is important and very much in society's interest that experimentation be permitted. We must have the ability to challenge the conventional wisdom. I think that we must not forget that there is a whole web of mechanisms here involved. There are not only the ones recently set up, hospital committees and the rest. There are malpractice decisions. There is some legislation. There is the question of due care in case law. There is a whole web of things here that can serve to regulate and keep some balance in such a type of thing.

As far as the first man to not radiate the thymus is concerned, I would point out what I said earlier about random selection. Many of the things that have gotten into our present practice and are not getting out of it were brought into it by chance-selected trials, anticoagulants and myocardial infarction, if you will. I mean they now have to be brought out of it again. But what we must have is the ability to challenge the conventional wisdom and discard therapies of no importance. Insofar as tonsillectomy is concerned, if I could dream up an experiment, a chance trial with indicators of measurement here, I would do that. I would be all for it.

THOMAS: I want only to say that these are not new problems for medicine. I suppose we have had variants of the tonsillectomy issue stretching back through all the millennia of our existence -- bleeding, cupping, and purging being only part of it. We do acquire habits that we institutionalize, and they are very hard to shake off. It would be my hope that now in these decades we could get into this sort of thing and perhaps then get out rather more directly, using more scientific methods than we have used in the past. One senses that hazards lie ahead of us and that they have got to be looked out for.

I would just add to the anticoagulant coronary problems that Dr. McDermott mentioned. During the period when anticoagulants were very widely and universally in use for this disease, they did cause problems of malpractice and lawsuits and the like. We are now engaged in discussions as to whether to apply antihypertensive therapy to all detectable hypertensives in our society, all the millions of them. I am not sure that any of us has foreseen either the benefits or the hazards of that, and this is going to have to be sorted through.

The tonsillectomy in our study became a rite of passage. It occurs to me that at the other end of life the coronary bypass surgery is another rite of passage, fortunately not passage in the direction that some of us had anticipated.

It must be said that there is a certain amount of fecklessness involved in these muddled experiences in which we find ourselves. There are ways of doing these things better. I would not object to regulations at a federal level in the sources from which the funds derive, either for paying for patient care or for paying for the research. They would continue to come, as they have been coming, out of HEW. I don't find any of them too egregious to live with. I would hate to see them bureaucratized and made something as complex and Byzantine as the regulations that have existed in past decades in FDA. This, it seems to me, would pose the almost certain hazard of having clinical research grind to a standstill in this country. We would only move forward when everyone was so possessed of a conviction of absolute certainty that the research itself would be uninteresting and probably not very important to do. But I think that the problem that we face from here on out -- the one that Mr. Gorovitz brought out -- is terribly important. I have no intention, and I am sure my colleagues have no intention, of trying to sweep it away or pretend that it does not exist. It does exist. It is an occasion for your heart to sink every time you think about it.

If regulations are necessary in order to provide the public with a condition where this sort of thing is not going to happen, I, for one, would not be opposed to it.

WILLARD GAYLIN: I would like to return to a line of questioning, one started by Dr. Hiatt and Dr. Sabin, and continued by Professor Gorovitz, because I don't think it was addressed adequately.

Dr. Moore started us off with a cultural history of experimentation that was inspirational in quality and the kind that drove me to apply to medical school. On getting into medical school, I met Carl Wiggers, a professor of physiology who notified us that medical intervention had probably cost more lives than it had saved. Well, I am not sure. I would have to leave it to your documentation committe whether that statement was accurate in 1947 when Dr. Wiggers made it. If there were more time I would ask Dr. Moore to spend ten minutes to balance his half hour by discussing those areas of medical experimentation that were either self-indulgent, insensitive, costly of human valuse, reducing of human dignity, or nonpurposive.

I would point to some of the recent work of Henry Beecher, who is dealing with those institutions with which Dr. Moore has a firsthand familiarity, and I am sure his knowledge of history goes beyond these more current days. Then I would like to ask the speakers as a group, granting the fact that government intervention can be harmful, where they would see some regulation of experimentation necessary. I would like each member to direct himself to where he feels the want of some regulation, if at all, and if not at all, I would like to hear that, too.

ROBBINS: I think the question you asked Dr. Moore in regard to the abuses is similar to one he was asked before. I will take a brief crack at that, because there is the classical series of horror stories, some of which are true horror stories. I suppose the one that has been most widely quoted was the syphilis experiment from Tuskegee. One can go back in history and identify many others. But I also would like to point out that some of the so-called horror stories that are ingrained in the conventional wisdom of people who talk about these things are not necessarily horror stories. Although they are horror stories to some and not horror stories to others, one will hear the litany. The Willowbrook experiments appear in most presentations on the subject of abuses. But yet one can find rational people, moral and ethical people who will support those experiments; and you will find moral and ethical people who will not. It is not a clearcut horror story.

I think there are many other abuses, some of which fall in the area of the kinds of surgery for changing people, such as lobotomies and things of this sort. I suspect in many instances these are quite unchallengeable horror stories. But I think there is a tendency, once somebody has challenged an experiment, to ingrain the story in the conventional wisdom and to simply repeat it. It almost comes into the range of gossip, and I think that that is a very unfortunate matter.

There is not time to enter into this topic in great detail, but I would like now to let each of the panelists make a closing statement addressing what has come up here.

McDERMOTT: I would simply like to close by stating, as I have before, that the risks involved are of every kind that any sort of a medical intervention can take. The dark side basically has to do with the fact that one person put another person into risk. How we meet the societal needs and still protect a certain amount of the individual's rights is something that is not clear to me. I say "certain amount of the individual's rights," because any other way of doing it is to take the position that the social good is the sum of all individual goods, and I simply do not think that proposition can stand up. It particularly cannot stand up in terms of what has been accomplished with society by research.

I became very interested, as all of us have in this business, in looking into the various writings, and particularly the *Social Contract* of Jean Jacques Rousseau, who certainly studied the questions of individual rights versus social rights. I discovered that he had intended to write a large textbook on this subject and that he had to settle for the intital essay because he could not figure his way out.

THOMAS: It has been my own experience in the last several years that the committees now mandated to exist within hospital centers for the review of all aspects of human experimentation seem to work very well in the environment that I am familiar with. This is not enough, I am sure, to satisfy all critics, but it needs to be said that the mechanism works very well. One way of telling that it works very well is that the quality of the research is obviously being scrutinized by more people within the institution qualified to do this. The institution, as an institution, now achieves responsibilities for all the research within its walls, which it was not aware of as a responsibility in the years before we drifted in this altogether desirable direction. I have no objection to seeing that mandated and stipulated in more regulations and to have the outcome be that the institution would assume all kinds of responsibility for human experimentation within its walls. I would not have any great objection to having people representing the patient population at large taking an active role in this kind of committee work.

McDERMOTT: You and I are licensed to practice medicine and surgery in the state of New York.

THOMAS: This is true. I have never taken out a tonsil in my life.

McDERMOTT: You were prevented somehow.

THOMAS: Yes. The second thing I wanted to say is simply to reiterate that I am not sure that there are very many issues with human experimentation confronting us today that I would regard as very important for mankind's future. I don't think that there is that much very interesting crucial research going on at this moment. There will be, however, and I think we should preserve the possibility of clinical research going on for at least the next century. One by one the major diseases that worry mankind and that give us the trouble, that give us heart sink when we think about what goes on inside a hospital, these are going to come down as we acquire more and more understanding of underlying mechanisms. This means cancer and heart disease and stroke and rheumatoid arthritis and even, as Dr. Sabin remarked, schizophrenia. And I hope we can preserve the system, faulty as it may be, so that when the occasion arises for making a frontal approach on, say, rheumatoid arthritis or schizophrenia, we can do these things and get the answers that I think then will turn out to be of great benefit to mankind at large.

DORIS HAIRE: I am President of the American Foundation for Maternal and Child Health. We have just done a national survey of state regulations regarding the retention and preservation of medical records. In the state of New York, a hospital can throw away records at the end of six years. Nurses' notes can be thrown out at the end of the hospital stay. This is valuable information that researchers should have, and I am stunned that New York would allow this to be destroyed.

MOORE: I would just like to take my turn on this closing bit to say that my response to Dr. Gorovitz and to Dr. Gaylin is affirmative: we should look at that, Dr. Beecher is sitting right there. He helped us to think more clearly about this with his work several years ago. And there is a little point there where I disagree with Dr. McDermott, in that I think there is a dark side. There is a dark side that is more than just people putting someone else at risk, and I just mentioned one or two egregious examples. I won't go into them any further. But there have been others, such as the tremendous wave of cardiac transplantations in 1968 and 1969, done without adequate immunosuppression and without adequate animal work. I think in each one of these things that it would be profitable to analyze the anatomy of those dark experiences and try to find out why they were that way.

ROBBINS: Thank you very much. I apologize to anyone who did not get a chance to speak this time. I hope you will later.

INDIVIDUAL RISKS vs. SOCIETAL BENEFITS

What Consent Is Needed?

INTRODUCTION TO THE CASES

Renée C. Fox

This Academy Forum is based on the premise that the social, legal, moral, and metaphysical issues associated with human experimentation confront us with a series of complex dilemmas that are neither easily nor properly resolved by simple value affirmations. Research with human beings that is at once ethical and feasible must be mindful of the potential risks and benefits that it entails for the individuals who are directly or indirectly involved in the investigative process, and for the larger societal community to which they and all of us belong. Some kind of dynamic equilibrium between the promises and perils of research, and between individual and societal considerations should ideally be struck -- an equilibrium that does not immoderately embolden investigators and their subjects, unduly fetter them, or relegate them to an irresolute state of limbo. I am tempted here to be somewhat aphoristic and say that it is far easier to recommend such a golden balance than it is to attain it.

Within this general framework, the cases on which the Forum program is built focus on the relationship between rigorous and responsible research with human subjects, the quality of their consent, and the equity of the way in which experimental advantages and risks are distributed among different individuals and groups. In these connections we will be particularly concerned with the fetus and the child, the military, the prisoner, and the poor. The identity of the human fetus, the immaturity of the child, the captivity of the prisoner, the chain of command to which the soldier is subject, and the deprivation of the poor all raise questions about whether their participation in research can be noncoercive, free of exploitation, knowledgeable, meaningful, and fair.

It has become almost a truism to affirm that informed voluntary consent is central to the ethicality of all research conducted with human

60

subjects. The litany-like ring of this statement is not only attributable to the essentiality of consent, but also to the frequency with which incantations to its importance have been made in the growing number of organized discussions and publications dealing with the ethics of human experimentation. Problems of distributive justice and equity are also being debated -- less frequently than problems of consent, perhaps, and more in connection with the allocation of scarce resources in the delivery of medical care than with regard to human experimentation.

Why is so much concerned interest in these kinds of issues being expressed? In part, this seems to be a collective, cumulative reaction to various kinds of abuses that have occurred in research with human subjects. Some diminution of generalized trust in the motivation, commitment, and competence of physicians appears to be involved here as well, and with it a lesser willingness to accept claims to autonomy and self-regulation made by the medical profession. Awed apprehension about some of the biomedical prospects that loom before us is also contributing to this interest: actual and anticipated developments in genetic engineering; life-support systems; birth technology; population control; the implantation of human, animal, and artificial organs; and the modification of human thought and behavior.

In a recent article[1] I have suggested that the preoccupation with human experimentation is part of a broader and deeper societal concern with ethical and existential issues related to biomedical progress and to the delivery of medical care. I have also observed that some of the same questions of values, beliefs, and meaning that have been raised with respect to medical research and care are occurring in other domains of American society. I have hypothesized that this convergence of moral and metaphysical themes may be part of a ramifying process of social and cultural change that is carrying American society toward a new stage of modernity, one in which we are joining scientific-technical and religious-philosophical issues that we used to separate. This rapprochement is graphically illustrated by the cases before us this afternoon: biomedical and behavioral research with the fetus and with the child.

However medical, legal, or sociological our starting point may be, somehow, in February of 1975, these considerations will inexorably lead us to ponder ethical and existential questions as well. What is life? When does it begin? What do we mean by viable life? When does a fetus acquire "protectable humanity"[2] or personhood? Who is the child? What identity, rights, and obligations does a child have independently of his or her biological or social parents? Should the balance of risks and benefits to which a child is subjected be any different from that deemed appropriate for an adult? Is there any morally indubitable way in which proper consent for experimentation on fetuses or children can be obtained? From whom should such consent be sought? From the would-have-been mother and/or father of the fetus? From the parents of the child? From the child himself? From a special surrogate designated by the society to represent new life?

As our discussions unfold, I invite you to consider my hypothesis: that the raising of such moral and metaphysical questions at a scientific forum like this one is part of a much larger happening, with long-range implications for the fundamental value and belief structures of our society.

If I may I would like to add a kind of postlude to those remarks that I have prepared, which grows out of my attentive appreciation of the remarks that were made this morning. It seemed to me that a common thread that ran through the presentations was the wistful entreaty that strictly biomedical issues associated with human experimentation ought ideally to be kept distinct from ethical, legal, political, social, and what I have called existential phenomena that also accompany these issues.

My own perspective on this is that the current reality situation precludes the achievement of this goal, whose desirability I also question. The kind of sociologically aseptic conditions that have been invoked do not currently exist empirically. In fact, as I have suggested, biological, medical, sociolegal, sociopolitical, and inherently religious questions are occurring in complex interaction with one another. And a whole series of social actors, not only biologists and medical professionals, but also ethicists, theologians, clergymen, lawyers, judges, congressmen, politicians, social scientists, government agencies, and various organized and unorganized groups of citizens, including juries, are already active participants in this process.

The problem then, it seems to me, is not so much to deplore this, but to deal adequately and creatively with it. Here we come to what seems to me to be one of the overarching questions to which this Forum ought to address itself. Can this conjuncture of issues be competently handled in the name of the entire society by anyone or even by the congeries of existing institutional complexes, be they the biomedical community, the polity, the courts of our land, or our clergy and philosophers? Or do we need a newly invented kind of social mechanism to deal with these issues?

In concluding, I would like to cite the Roe vs. Wade decision on the legality of abortion and the repercussions of that case in recent weeks. In that particular decision handed down by the Supreme Court, Associate Justice Blackmun, in summarizing the majority opinion, indicated that he felt it was unseemly for justices of a court to rule on the question of when does life begin, and that we would have to wait upon ethicists, theologians, biologists, and the like for the answer to that very complex and awesome question. Yet, it seems to me inescapably that in ruling at all on abortion, one does tackle covertly, if not overtly, that question, because in that particular decision, of course, a distinction was made between the first and second trimesters of pregnancy. I cannot think of any legal position that could be taken on that question which would not blatantly, if not manifestly, get into some of these issues-- issues that some of us would like to be able to clear from the landscape so that we could deal more straightforwardly, perhaps, with the strictly biomedical features of the phenomena before us.

THE FETUS

Charles A. Alford, Jr.
Frederick C. Battaglia
Robert B. Jaffe
Audrey K. Brown
Elizabeth D. Hay

CHARLES ALFORD

Aside from discussing the pros and cons of various categories of human
research, this meeting also focuses on life as a dynamic process. In
keeping with this concept, it seems appropriate that the opening case
session should focus on the initial stages of this process, namely
embryonic life.

The ethical, legal, social, medical, and scientific issues posed by
research on the human fetus are far more complex than some of those to
be discussed in the other sessions. The reasons for this are many.
Some are obvious; others less so.

Consider, for instance, that research in this area involves not just
an individual, but at least three persons: an unseen patient, the
fetus; the mother; and the father. Therefore, the central issue of
informed consent and who might be permitted to give it is a critical
problem in need of resolution in the immediate future.

Recent decisions of the Supreme Court relaxing legal controls on
abortion, and the violent reactions of various segments of our society
to these decisions, make the task of this particular panel difficult if
not frightening. We all unanimously agree, however, that the enormous
problems and the debates surrounding modern abortion laws should not
become so overwhelming as to preclude fetal research, either that ongoing or that projected for the future. For if this would happen, it
would herald a medical tragedy unparalleled in modern times.

Even total cessation of human fetal research would not change the
abortion rates in this country to any significant degree, since no form
of research is a major stimulus to their presumed increasing numbers.
Instead, ablation of fetal research would hamper proper medical care

for millions of innocent pregnant women not comtemplating abortion and most particularly for their babies whether born or unborn.

Simply stated, modern medical research, development, and practice are so inextricably linked, especially in the areas of obstetrics and pediatrics encompassed by fetal research, that a deterrent to the human aspect would be immediately translated into reduced medical care for untold numbers of young infants and their mothers. That this possibility could become a reality in a civilized society is unthinkable, truly inexcusable, no matter how important the real or imagined issues might be that allow it to come into being.

As combined practitioners, academicians, and researchers, mandated through our various professions to protect the health and well-being of pregnant women and their children and to guarantee their rights for even greater future improvements, this panel views the fetus as a critical link in the continuum of life. But to provide maximum medical care for the protection of the fetus, we must better understand its normal development, the deviations from norm that lead to disease, and the causes for these deviations. Without this knowledge, the necessary steps toward intrauterine therapy, either now or tomorrow, become impossible. The path to becoming a realistic physician to the fetus will be strewn with one ethical stumbling block after another. This is a necessary outcome because of our ignorance and the resulting mystique surrounding it. We accept the challenge of solution, and look forward to the improvements of tomorrow, no matter how difficult the task may seem today.

From this point on, we would like to present our view of what fetal research is all about, and essentially it will come in three units. Dr. Battaglia, first, will introduce the subject and attempt to categorize for you our view of what is entailed under the subject of fetal research and to identify those areas that involve the greatest ethical issues. The second will be an overview, from the obstetrical standpoint, by Dr. Jaffe. Finally there will be an overview from the pediatric standpoint by Dr. Audrey Brown. Dr. Hay will then add comments before the discussion.

FREDERICK BATTAGLIA

I would like to begin by stressing very briefly what I do not intend to dwell on, namely, the use of living tissues from dead fetuses or from their placentas, because I think for most of us this does not present any major ethical dilemmas. Leroy Walters has written recently about this, using some analogies that I think bring up some ethical issues even in this area. But I think for most of us involved in biomedical research, we see little problem with the use of living tissues from dead organisms.

I would stress at the start, because this does get somewhat confusing, that I am referring here to a nonliving organism. That is quite different from a previable fetus, in which viability, for me at least, is a definition of a future prognosis -- that is, will you live one month, one week, one day -- whereas we can decide what is or is not living at this instant in time, and define a biologic state. In the use of living tissues from dead fetuses, from their placentas, we have an area where a great deal of exciting work has gone on in cell biology and virology, and where we are not presented, I think, with major ethical dilemmas.

So, I would like to move on to the more difficult area, and that is the question of research on living fetuses and abortuses, whether or not we make a prognosis that they are viable over a given length of time. Here, of course, we have a number of difficulties. First of all, there are the arguments that such research in man is absolutely essential and must go on. Most of the time this case is made on the basis of differences between species, differences that would preclude our obtaining useful information from animal research that could then be applied to man. I think there are legitimate examples of this, which Dr. Jaffe and other members of the panel will stress.

Again, to give balance to our program, I would say that while some of the scientists may have had different experiences, my own has been that as I have reviewed protocols aimed at such research on living fetuses or living abortuses, the experimental design often has not adequately reflected the current state of the field. The considerable body of data that has been collected, demonstrating the marked differences in physiology and biochemistry introduced by studying fetuses at different gestational ages or under different conditions of stress even within the same species, is often overlooked. Thus, strictly on a scientific basis, these protocols would not be acceptable, in that the experimental design precludes obtaining definitive answers.

However, even assuming high quality of experimental design and the importance of the questions posed for solution -- which gets us into the realm of cost-benefit ratios, and which to me is a minimum criteria for human research, not an end in itself -- I still believe that all such research on living fetuses and living abortuses would take us into the realm of a discussion of some kind of informed consent, by whatever groups or individuals.

In general, my guidelines would be similar to those one would use, in most instances, in evaluating the appropriateness of research protocols on infants and children. The research could be considered in two categories, as some of the speakers have already done: namely, a category where we are discussing research that is without risk or harm to the fetus, and another where there is a degree of risk involved.

In the first category, given the above approval, my concern would be to allow such researchers as much latitude as possible. That is, it need not be therapeutic or immediately relevant to this fetus or to those parents, but could be directed at helping prenatal biology and medicine to progress in a more general context. Such research might include, for instance, collecting umbilical cord blood samples or urine samples for analyses of pesticides or whatever. However, I would stress that we could insist that the best technical advice be brought to bear on the review of the protocol. Again, the idea being to reduce the number of different studies required to answer the same or related questions.

In this area, I might mention the obvious problem that physicians take care of patients, and that the M.D. degree in itself does not ensure any certification or qualification for research. It is true, in general, that animal research and basic research are expensive, and thus require funding from granting agencies, which take them into a peer review system. That may not be true, although granted it is a very small percentage I am referring to here, but it need not necessarily be true of all human research. The fact that the accreditation groups that are coming along -- as well as subspecialty boards in maternal-fetal medicine, in neonatal-perinatal medicine -- may also now insist on research credentials exaggerates the problem. The increased emphasis on primary care teaching in medical schools, and the need for a growing body of service-oriented, teaching-oriented physicians, again, brings up problems in review of human research protocols that are especially relevant to the area we are discussing today. Where an area of biology moves ahead rapidly, there may be comparatively few numbers of faculty at each school to review such protocols.

So, again, I think we could all agree as a general principle that the research protocols on humans should adhere to the highest possible scientific standards and introduce through one mechanism or another more required consultation and advice from appropriate scientists into protocol design.

If we come back to the group then, where we are considering research in which some degree of risk is involved, again I would feel that one should be sure that the risk to the fetus or abortus should not be life-threatening in and of itself -- that is, the research protocol should not in itself preclude survival -- and that the research should have the potential at least for being therapeutic to the pregnancy, mother or fetus.

In general, the ethical practices with regard to fetal research that I would follow are similar to those provided in the Peel Report and so elegantly presented in Paul Ramsey's recent book on the ethics of fetal research. Additionally, I think that there should be some firm definition by some governmental agencies beyond which research on the living abortus becomes considered in the same light as the living new-born infant. By definition I mean something we can hang onto by weight or gestation. This definition should be a firm one, since it is essentially an attempt at delineating viability -- that is, a prognosis of continued survival with full recognition of the errors inherent in physician judgment of gestational age and of the markedly different neonatal prognosis of infants of the same size but different ages.

Again I would return to looking at mechanisms that would not be-labor us with organization, but at the same time would tighten up the protocol and the input from a variety of scientists into human research.

Finally, I would reemphasize the fact that the research conducted on living tissues from dead fetuses and on placental tissue, for most of us at least, presents little ethical dilemma and it represents the area that has been tapped and used so successfully in cell biology and virology.

ROBERT JAFFE

There are many avenues by which the broad area called fetal research might be approached. The approach that I should like to take is to discuss this research in the context of first, those advances in medical care that would have been proscribed had such research not been permitted in the past; and second, some problems in medical care for which present and future fetal investigation may provide some solutions.

Before embarking on this discussion, it might be well to review and define briefly those various areas that have been grouped under the heading of fetal research. There is minimal disagreement about the conduct of research in some of these areas, and more active discussion of others. These definitions include the distinctions between use of dead versus living material; the use of individual tissues as contrasted with the study of the whole organism; the distinction between previable (or nonviable) and viable fetuses; and the utilization of the fetus in research as contrasted with use of other tissues resulting from pregnancy, including the placenta, fluids, and membranes.

There are two documents that have dealt most extensively with these issues, and I shall use them, in part, in framing these distinctions. These documents are the report of the advisory group to the Department of Health and Social Security in the United Kingdom, chaired by Sir John Peel, on the use of fetuses and fetal material for research; and the proposed guidelines for the protection of special subjects in biomedical research, promulgated by an advisory group of the Department of Health, Education, and Welfare here in the United States.

The Peel report defines fetal death as the state in which the fetus shows none of the signs of life and is incapable of being made to function as a self-sustaining whole. As Dr. Battaglia mentioned, individuals of many persuasions feel that research on the dead fetus should be permitted to continue and does not require restrictions or legislation.

Secondly, the distinction should be made between the fetus as an intact organism for study, and the study of individual tissues. Sir John Peel's group found that in most instances fetal tissues were used, rather than the whole organism, as tissues and cells may continue to live for a period after the fetus itself has died, even if they are separated from it.

Additionally, the distinction should be made between the study of the fetus and the study of other products of conception including the placenta, fluids, and membranes. Few would maintain that study of these products is at issue.

We come, then, to the distinction between the previable and viable fetus. There is no definition of viability that is satisfactory to all, and comprehensive analysis of the definition is beyond the scope and time constraints of this presentation. A commission established by recent congressional legislation will address this issue extensively. The Peel Report defines a viable fetus as one that has reached the stage of maintaining the coordinated operation of its component parts so that is is capable of functioning as a self-sustaining whole and independently of any connection with the mother. The proposed policy of the Department of Health, Education, and Welfare maintains that the presence of the beating heart is not, of itself, proof of viability, and that an additional prerequisite be the capacity for expansibility of the lungs. I would concur that the presence of a beating heart alone is not an acceptable criterion for defining viability either of the fetus or of the adult. I might suggest additionally that medical practices resulting from previous and current fetal research have permitted a redefinition of the age and weight of the previable fetus and the viable fetus.

Having made these distinctions, let me now consider some of those areas of medical care to which fetal research in the past has contributed and some of those areas in which present and future investigation might be expected to make inroads. Parenthetically, I might add that much of this investigation has been of excellent caliber and conducted by well-trained investigators, while some research dealing with human subjects, just as research dealing with animal models, has been less than optimal. One should not abandon needed research because investigations in an area have not been carried out in an optimal fashion by ideal investigators.

Among those areas of maternal, child, and general medical care that have benefited by fetal research are:

1. the modern management and prevention of Rh blood group sensitization

2. the antenatal detection of fetal metabolic and genetic abnormalities by sampling the amniotic fluid that surrounds the unborn fetus in the uterus

3. the development of vaccines for the prevention of several viral diseases

4. the assessment of fetal lung maturity by chemical tests performed on the amniotic fluid

5. improvements in the prevention and treatment of prematurity, the leading cause of neonatal mortality

6. hormonal measurements performed on the mother's blood or urine, which serve as valuable reflections of the status of the unborn fetus.

68

I should like to elaborate on work that has been carried out in each
of these areas.

The contemporary diagnosis, management, and now prevention of
isoimmunization of the infant of the Rh negative mother represents a
remarkable epoch in medicine. Many unborn babies were sensitized
because of immune, antigen-antibody reactions leading to severe, often
fatal, anemia in utero. Important strides were made in the prenatal
diagnosis of this disorder by obtaining a sample of amniotic fluid.
The amount of blood breakdown pigments in the fluid was found to corre-
late well with the severity of the baby's anemia. When the degree of
anemia was so severe that the fetuses would otherwise have died while
still in the uterus, it was found that they could be transfused while
still in the intrauterine environment. Intrauterine transfusion
initially was an experimental procedure, which could not have been
assessed completely in animals and which has resulted in the salvage of
a number of previously helpless infants. Subsequently, by further
experimental studies in humans, it was found that this disease process
could be prevented by the administration of immune globulin. Thus,
through the use of experimental procedures involving pregnant women and
their unborn fetuses, the diagnosis, management, and subsequent prevention of a frequently fatal disease evolved.

The use of amniotic fluid obtained during the course of pregnancy
has led to another group of advances in medical management. Utilizing
fluid obtained from the uterus of the pregnant woman for specific
chromosomal and biochemical studies, a number of genetic and metabolic
disorders can be diagnosed early in pregnancy. One such disorder is
mongolism, which frequently is associated with mental retardation. Had
the previously experimental procedure of amniocentesis, that is,
obtaining a sample of the amniotic fluids surrounding the fetus by
insertion of a needle into the pregnant woman's uterus, been proscribed,
these advances would not have been possible.

Another area in which advances have been made is virology and immunology. Several investigators were awarded Nobel prizes for work using
fetal tissues that led to the development of vaccines, the administration of which prevent polio and measles. Without the use of these
tissues from aborted fetuses, this work would have been hampered
significantly.

One of the major challenges to contemporary obstetrics and pediatrics
is prematurity, a major cause of neonatal death and morbidity. The premature infant has difficulty largely because of respiratory distress.
Performing experimental studies on fetal lungs has led to increased
understanding of the development of the surface active agent that
enables the lung to function properly. Using fluid obtained by amniocentesis, it is now possible to measure the compounds involved in the
formation of this surface active agent, and thereby to assess the degree
of fetal lung maturation. This information is of extreme value to the
obstetrician in several clinical situations, including the determination
of the optimal time for delivery of the infant of the diabetic mother.

These determinations also enable the obstetrician to alert the pediatrician of the impending delivery of an infant who will develop respiratory distress so that preparation for appropriate therapeutic measures can be made.

Turning to the area of endocrinology, hormone formation, metabolism, and function differ markedly between other animal species, including monkeys, and humans. Basic knowledge resulting from experimental studies in humans of the formation and metabolism of hormones in pregnancy has led to clinical tests to assess the well-being of certain high-risk pregnancies.

In addition, ultimately there is no adequate way to assess the safety of drugs, including antibiotics, which we use to treat pregnant women and their offspring other than to study the efficacy, safety, and metabolism of these drugs in the groups of women and children for whom they are intended. These studies must include adequate controls, that is, subjects who do not have the disease process for which the particular drug is intended. In fact, all meaningful scientific studies require adequate controls. For example, to understand the abnormality of intrauterine growth retardation of the fetus, we must study normal patterns of intrauterine growth.

Having discussed some areas in which various types of fetal research have had an impact upon advances in medical care -- advances that would not have been possible had such work been proscribed previously -- I should like to direct my attention to a few of those areas in which present and future research can reasonably be expected to lead to improvements in care of pregnant women and their offspring.

While strides have been made in the diagnosis and management of the premature infant, prematurity, with its attendant lung problems, remains a leading cause of newborn mortality and infant morbidity. Further studies of normal and abnormal lung maturation may be expected to lead to further improvements in the prevention as well as management of these problems.

When the factors responsible for the initiation of labor in women are known, a more intelligent approach to the prevention of premature labor may be effected. Already medications are being studied in pregnant women that appear to hold great promise in preventing premature labor. It has been reasonably well established that those factors responsible for the onset of labor in certain experimental animals are strikingly different from the causes of labor in women. While animal studies can and should pave the way for studies in humans, ultimately information obtained in animal studies must be translated into information for humans. This can only be done by studies of both normal and altered physiologic states.

Additionally, knowledge of normal function of the heart and blood vessels during human development should lead to a greater understanding of congenital heart disease and conceivably of heart disease manifest later in life.

Finally, in a more speculative vein, there are good reasons to believe that information obtained concerning the endocrinology and

immunology of pregnancy may be relevant to an understanding of basic
mechanisms involved in cancer development. Without meaning to sound
melodramatic, if improvements in maternal care, infant health and survival, congenital and acquired heart disease, prevention of certain
viral diseases, and inroads into understanding basic mechanisms in
cancer and immune mechanisms can be effected by well-structured, carefully conducted research in the pregnant woman and the fetus, it would
seem rational to further and foster this research now and in the future.

AUDREY BROWN

I am glad that today we find obstetricians and pediatricians agreeing
so well that our speeches are almost identical. However, I will have
to deviate initially from my prepared statement, because I think the
thread that inspired Dr. Jaffe's speech and perhaps a little of mine
was a bit different than what was touched upon this morning. When we
are discussing fetal and neonatal research, and particularly research
in the living fetus, I think both of us are reacting to the possibility
that not only is society asking that research be improved and that the
frivolous research be eliminated, but there is a real threat that without understanding the contributions of research on the living fetus,
there may be a real movement to ban all research. That focuses the
question quite differently than the general subject of research in
human subjects.

The other definition that Dr. Jaffe did not touch upon is the one of
research itself. It is a word that I am sure means many things to many
people in this room. But I have read definitions of research as applied
to human beings, and it is frightening to me to realize that anything
innovative or not established by common practice or a series of experiments is considered in the broad term of research. Those of us who are
dealing with an entirely new possibility, fetal medicine, or the sal-
vaging of the lives of the premature, face that definition with a great
deal of trepidation, because nothing we have done in the past has
worked. Are we to continue then to try to do nothing new? If research
in those terms is banned, we are in great difficulty.

It is our purpose today to discuss means by which we can assure
protection to human subjects, including the fetus and newborn, who are
involved with us in the pursuit of information that may contribute to
better health care for the fetus and for the infant. We can assume,
and indeed it has been documented, that physicians offering new and
advanced treatment are, in the main, acting in good faith, and that
the majority of medical research meets the highest ethical standards.
Societal concern is directed toward developing means by which protection
of all subjects at all times is assured -- an ideal situation -- while
at the same time giving assurance that knowledge and potential cures
will and can continue to be sought. We must be certain, as Dr. Fox
pointed out, to balance these two objectives, lest we deny to this and

to future generations their right to hope for cures of disorders that are presently unconquered.

The particular problem which I am to address is the perplexing one concerning the need for further knowledge of fetal and neonatal disorders, because it is this area that has been left untouched for generations. We are beginning to realize that we have the obligation to be true physicians to the fetus. The problem requiring our attention is to assure the possibility of investigation involving the fetus and newborn in order to continue to develop means of care for the fetus, while at the same time taking into account the rights of that fetus and the newborn.

Most of the advances in fetal medicine are new. They have occurred certainly within the past fifteen years because of the realization that the fetus was indeed a patient, one who often had been denied the possibility of being born because of his relative inaccessibility to treatment prior to birth. In the past, physicians would only wait to treat the fetus after he was in view, after he was born. But now we know that this inaccessibility -- and a bit of our own stupidity -- does not allow us to disclaim the responsibility for his direct care.

The major event that initiated direct treatment of the fetus came from the courageous effort of Dr. Liley of New Zealand, who realized that the fetus, doomed to die in the uterus with severe anemia caused by Rh hemolytic disease, was only two inches away from a possible life-saving blood transfusion. Although these two inches of the mother were a physical barrier, they really represented more of a conceptual barrier. The frustrated physician realized that this barrier could be breached by a needle, reaching from the extrauterine into the intra-uterine world. He could offer life-saving blood if only he were permitted to reach into this sanctum sanctorum. With the first transfusion, a fetus was saved from certain death, and because of Dr. Liley's willingness and courage to try this new approach, that life and now many other lives of the unborn have been preserved.

The success of that effort opened up an entirely new era of hope and of responsibility for physicians to the fetus. And the treatment of Rh hemolytic disease of the unborn is not the only disorder of the fetus that can be diagnosed and treated while the fetus is still in utero alive. We have come to realize that many fetal disorders can be detected in utero, including infections and inherited disorders. We do not yet have any idea how many of them might be treated there, and how many disabilities might readily be stopped or prevented right then.

To find these answers and to extend health care to the fetus, new approaches must be found. Since these inevitably involve the mother very directly, is her consent enough? Is her refusal enough to deny him this hope of life? For the larger question that we face today, can society take on the burden through legislation of denying the mother the freedom of such decision to try to save her child, if her child can only be saved through what in the broad sense of the word is research?

As a pediatrician, let me take a few minutes to indicate how essential it is that the fetus and the newborn continue to be studied if we are to save lives that are presently assumed to be lost. While there must, of course, be continued vigilance against abuse, every effort should be made to encourage, rather than to discourage, innovative approaches to these old problems. Many of the problems bridging fetal and neonatal life center upon prematurity. Why is an infant born early? How can we keep him alive even though physiologically he may not yet be ready for our world and to live in air? And there is the very large problem of when do we offer him every medical advance in order that he may survive? Does society by limiting experimentation in effect deny these infants their right to live? How many of the disabilities of the premature long thought to be inherent in being born too soon are actually preventable if only we knew more? What is the magnitude of this problem?

There are more than 3 million infants born each year in this nation. About one quarter million are of low birth weight, that is, they weigh less than 2,500 grams or 5 1/2 pounds. Some of these infants are true immature or premature infants and are born too soon. Others are deprived or suffering from infection before birth and are born too small and poorly developed, even though they are born at term. About one-fifth of the low-birth-weight group die before the end of the first month of extrauterine life. Among the survivors many will be afflicted with disease or disabilities. It has becom increasingly evident that we can markedly reduce the risk of both death and disability through intensive efforts and investigation.

Some disabilities one might even say are worse than death itself. They will be lifelong, and the child might have to be institutionalized at the cost of $5,000 per year. But some are truly related to the fact that very small immature infants have failed to receive the most intensive and sophisticated care required for their normal survival, for specialized care is still not available to all. But within the past fifteen years, application of new life support systems has proven that even immature infants can survive and live normal lives. Most of the systems are new and are still being improved under research programs directed toward perfecting intensive care. The techniques applied to these infants are very much like those we offer to adults so they might gain a few more years after a coronary. Only with regard to the premature, it is their fourscore years that we are trying to protect.

These techniques include special monitoring devices, automatic temperature control, respiratory ventilators, positive airway pressure devices, special lamps that reduce the risk of jaundice and concomitant brain damage. These intensive efforts to save the lives of the immature and to assure their normal development are threatened by well-motivated but ambiguously stated legislation that would ban research on living but nonviable fetuses. It could be claimed that these immature infants, whom we try to salvage, are truly previable or nonviable. It is true that without our dedicated help many could not survive. It is true that without new knowledge we cannot extend to them the hope of normal life. It must be realized by those posing such legislation that many immature babies, who would have been considered nonviable ten years ago, are now rather routinely saved and are alive thanks to fetal and neonatal research. Had restrictive legislation been passed ten years ago, these infants would still be considered nonviable, and they would in fact be dead.

Let me expand on some specific examples. More than half of the deaths that occur in the first week of life are due to respiratory failure, directly related to the inability of the immature infant to keep his lungs expanded and to breathe air. These infants have been doomed to die not because of congenital anomalies or disabilities or devastating infections, but because of a temporary inadequacy occurring because they were born too soon. Physicians who take care of the newborn have devoted their clinical and research efforts to analysis of this problem. Within the past ten years they have been able to understand why the premature infant was uniquely affected, and subsequently they have been able to reduce the death rate due to respiratory distress by almost 50 percent.

It is difficult to trace an idea in science. Thousands of attempts are made in medical research. Each success in some way furthers our ability to extend human life. The last few steps are giant ones; the first are often feeble and faltering. With regard to respiratory distress, it might surprise some of you to know that Maimonides in the twelfth century expanded the Talmudic concepts to include early detection of, and manual resuscitation for, sudden respiratory arrest in the newborn. That was not established practice then; it was an early research effort to improve the viability of the prematurely born.

Giant steps have been taken through fetal and neonatal research in the past few years, much of it postdating the publicized death of the last son of John Kennedy. Patrick Bouvier Kennedy died, as most premature infants die, with respiratory distress. Recent research involving the fetus has enabled the physician, as Dr. Jaffe pointed out, to identify the infant at risk before he is born by examining the amniotic fluid, looking for specific phospholipids that line the lung and make breathing possible. When these are not found, every effort is made to delay delivery until the lipids appear, indicating that the infant will be able to cope and to breathe and to survive in air.

Some infants cannot wait to be born. To keep such infants alive, new means of temporarily substituting for their inadequate respiratory efforts had to be developed. These new efforts employing sophisticated means of supplying continuous positive airway pressure have proven successful. Prior to 1968, 73 percent of infants with respiratory distress severe enough to require ventilation died. When it was shown that continuous pressure in the alveolus of the lung could substitute for the infant's failure to expand his own lung, mortality in the group who require ventilation has fallen dramatically. Now, even severely affected infants have a fifty-fifty chance of survival.

74

So, from the twelfth century to the late twentieth, we have come slowly to offer life to a significant number of affected infants. If the present pace of development of sophisticated life support systems is allowed to continue, we may be able to offer hope of survival to all such distressed infants. There are indications from even more recent investigative efforts that we may not only be able to forecast, but to prevent respiratory distress by administering drugs to the fetus that induce the development of the essential features of the lung prior to birth.

These exciting efforts extend real hope of life to the immature and to the presently previable. These infants cannot and could not be saved by established procedures. Effective therapy in the nursery today is, I am afraid, categorized as research, because it is all new. Only relatively recently have pediatricians been convinced that premature infants can develop normally. Only relatively recently has there been an appreciation of the fact that delivery of sophisticated and intensive care can not only save lives but prevent brain damage that so frequently is associated with premature birth. The realization that these immature infants are essentially good babies with a temporary inability to meet the challenge of life outside the womb, rather than infants doomed to be abnormal, has led to a remarkable new effort to support them during the period of adaptation. This has led to a reappraisal of the steps in fetal development and an effort to develop means of inducing early maturation of functions or substituting for it.

I speak then in support of innovative means of offering life to those presently considered nonviable, for within my own life as a physician I have seen a remarkable change in our ability to lower the age of viability. I also speak in support of innovative efforts to work together, as in this Forum, with other concerned members of society to develop the best possible means of preventing abuses in research on the fetus and newborn. The failure of present means and present ethical concepts to meet the conceptual challenges brought on by such rapid advances in the scientific aspects of these efforts does not, in my mind, constitute a reason to freeze the present state of our scientific knowledge. It should stimulate efforts to work together to develop the ethical framework in which to advance, while still protecting the rights of the human fetus and newborn. Some of these rights have been defined. Others have not. One key question bothering all of us today and that needs to be addressed is: Who shall have the right to deny the hope of life?

ELIZABETH HAY

I would just like to comment on the question of the value of doing research on fetuses from the point of view not of the clinician, which has been the issue so far, but from the point of view of the biologist and, if you will, of the woman.

75

Renée Fox has referred to the fact that we are in a changing society. Our values are changing. There is a need now for people to get together in all disciplines to discuss these problems. Not only are we changing our social world, but we are also changing nature's world. Nature at this moment is faced with a dilemma in terms of her way of solving evolution and the development and progression of the species. Man now has decided, certainly in this country and in many other countries, that the population for many reasons must become stable. In this country, it is, at this moment, stable. The average woman in this room will raise a family of two children. It is her right that these two children be as normal as possible. It is also nature's right, if the species is to carry on, that we do what we can to ensure that the fetuses born into this world will be normal.

INQUIRY AND COMMENTARY

LOIS SCHIFFER: I am an attorney at the Center for Law and Social Policy in Washington. I, in fact, quite strongly agree with most of what has been said here today, but would like to bring up one more point, which I think has not been dwelled on, although it has been alluded to by Dr. Jaffe. In considering fetal research, it is very important we think to take into account the interest of women, and particularly pregnant women, in setting up any controls that are going to be placed on fetal research and any procedures for its use.

Specifically, in a number of ways this matter comes to the fore. First of all, it really emphasizes the need to continue biomedical research on the fetus in order to develop methods for helping the pregnant woman, her nutrition and health. And, also, it is important that fetal research not be limited in any way that prevents the mother from partaking of therapy or treatment that will assist her health. For example, if a pregnant woman in the fourth month of her pregnancy determines that she has some kind of cancer, and only an experimental chemical will help her, there is no way that fetal research can legally be limited pursuant to the Supreme Court decisions to prevent her from undertaking that therapy.

We also think that fetal research must be undertaken in a way that gives the pregnant woman as full as possible control over her own health. Also, she should have the right to consent for herself rather than having paternal and spousal consent in any fetal research that is involved with pregnancy termination or experimentation that is focused on the woman's health and not the health of the fetus. We think this is particularly important because the NIH guidelines, which have been mentioned, specifically give both the father and the spouse a greater right, actually, than the fetus,

76

pursuant to the Supreme Court decision. This is simply not permissible.

Finally, we would say that when ethical committees and boards are established to take into account the problems of fetal research and to decide whether a particular research should go forward, it is very important that women be placed on these boards. Although men have certainly shown themselves to be sympathetic to the problems of women, there are many times when they simply cannot adequately represent those interests.

ROBBINS: Would anybody from the panel like to comment?

ALFORD: We agree.

RICHARD BEHRMAN: I have a specific question that I would be interested in hearing the panel discuss. Is there any situation in which an individual at low statistical risk should be subjected to a substantial risk from an experiment for the probable benefit of a larger group of which he is a part even though he or she is not likely to get a direct benefit? In answering that, would you consider a viable fetus as much an individual as an adult, and should the rule be the same for experimenting on that viable fetus versus the nonviable fetus? I think this is one of the central issues, to see what is similar and dissimilar among those three groups.

BATTAGLIA: I thought I got at that a bit, Dr. Behrman, because I made a distinction between two problems. One is working with previable or living fetuses. Then, within that category, I broke it down into research with and without risk. I said that when you enter the realm where there is risk involved, it seemed to me that you would need to have the potential for therapeutic research.

You will notice in Dr. Jaffe's list of the benefits of research, that they were not all research on the fetus, with the single exception of the intra-abdominal transfusions, and that was therapeutic. So I think I was trying to get at that issue, but perhaps did not present it clearly.

JAFFE: Without being able to answer that question, it is, I think, a central and very difficult one; and although I gave only one example, I suspect that there are others. At our institution, and I understand recently in Boston, the relatively new technique of getting at the fetus -- the so-called fetoscopy, in which an instrument is introduced that enables one to visualize the fetus in utero and get a sample of blood from that fetus -- has been stopped because of current concerns about fetal research. That technique enables one potentially to diagnose sickle cells. Although I mentioned one example of getting at the fetus -- and if proscriptions become strict enough that may be the only one example -- there are I think other horizons to which medical investigation is directing itself. These will also bear on research involving the fetus in utero and would lead to benefits either to that fetus and/or to the greater number of fetuses at which the research is aimed.

FRANZ INGELFINGER: I come from Massachusetts, a state that, according to the *Washington Post* this morning, is in disgrace. I want to lead on from that and ask the panel a fairly specific question, because that state is facing other problems, and except for Dr. Battaglia possibly, I have not heard any specific comments on them. There are several doctors who will be tried later this summer for having given antibiotics just preceding a planned abortion, with the purpose of studying the fetus after it has been aborted to determine how much of the antibiotic got into the fetal tissue.

This is, according to many of the Massachusetts legislators, research on a living fetus. I think, strictly speaking, it is. You are giving antibiotics to a living fetus, even though it will be a dead fetus in twenty-four hours. I would like to hear the panel commit themselves on this kind of research.

ALFORD: I think one comment that should be made concerns the mandate of the FDA and how they function with regard to the administration of drugs to pregnant women: this is, they must demonstrate that if a person is to introduce this drug it will not be harmful to the fetus. It has been clearly shown already that there are a lot of differences between the way almost any drug is handled by the mother and perhaps by the fetus, if it is even transmitted to the fetus. So essentially nothing could really be introduced for the pregnant woman, according to the mandate of the FDA, unless we can study both the mother and the fetus, because of the possible danger for one or the other in attempting to treat one or the other. Therefore, I see nothing wrong, at least philosophically, with the type of research that was being attempted in Boston.

JAFFE: I wonder, Dr. Ingelfinger, if we do not have to try and balance risks, too, here. Given the fetuses about which you were speaking -- those that were destined for abortion -- if one is attempting to use antibiotics in those fetuses not destined for abortion, might it be better to study the effects of antibiotics in the fetus to be aborted than to risk that study in fetuses that will not be?

I think these are very difficult and not easily solved questions. I think that the Forum members have probably addressed the questions that we have addressed through the eyes of our background and our information, that is, from a medical background. Perhaps it was one-sided from that point of view. I think those who have background and experience in dealing with ethical issues, in addition to physicians, must also have their input into this whole process. I am sure that Dr. Fox and her colleagues can make very meaningful

78

inputs into this. I think that in concert, perhaps, we can arrive at the guidelines for ethically based decisions on the fetus.

In a recent editorial a question was posed by Dr. Mary Ellen Avery, Professor of Pediatrics at Harvard, for which I do not know the answer. If a physician and a patient make a contract for an abortion -- and I think indeed that this should be an issue that is between the physician and the patient -- if the patient requests an abortion and the physician agrees to this abortion, and if that abortus is then larger than it was thought to be and so fulfills the criteria for viability, who makes the decision as to what to do with that fetus? It was not the wish of the mother for that fetus to be allowed to be viable. The physician is in a dilemma, and would really welcome help in making that decision. I do not know the answer.

ROBBINS: Dr. Brown, do you want to make a comment on this?

BROWN: I will avoid the last comment. I do not think anybody is prepared to answer. But with regard to Dr. Ingelfinger's question, there is another side that I have not heard and one in which I am interested as a mother.

I was interested in the concept that some girls seeking abortion had welcomed the opportunity to have meaningful research done rather than simply to lose an infant. Are we denying women some satisfaction, some contribution to society, if we should deny all research on abortuses or on those destined to be aborted? I would love to hear some of the women comment on that.

ALEXANDER CAPRON: I am from the University of Pennsylvania Law School. I have now three comments, very briefly, on the remark Dr. Ingelfinger just made.

The interesting thing, it seems to me, about the Massachusetts case is that the cooperative arrangement that Dr. Jaffe presupposed between the women and the doctors seems to have been absent and seems, in the case of the indictments there, to really have been the stumbling block, because at the time that that research went on, the Massachusetts statute on fetal research had not been passed, and no doctors had been charged with grave robbing.

If they had had the consent -- I don't mean to comment on the facts, for I am not aware of them beyond what appears in the press -- the Uniform Anatomical Gift Act allows the parents, in this case, to permit research on or the study of the dead fetuses to see if the erythromycin had passed, indeed, into them and where it was located in the body. So, had their been a cooperative arrangement between the maternal subjects and the doctors, that the research would have permitted that autopsy in that study, there probably would not be a basis for indictment, as far as I can see.

I wanted to raise a question for Dr. Battaglia and Dr. Jaffe, who used this concept of viability. It is a very attractive idea

for distinguishing between groups of fetal subjects. In part, as
Ms. Schiffer mentioned, the Supreme Court has used that as a bright
line separating those women who can have abortions and those who
only can have them with very grave restrictions. I wonder, however,
why we are going to use viability and if we are clear about why we
think viability is a useful concept in the case of fetal research.

One thing that viability does is to tell us those fetuses that
are in need of intensive care and have a good chance for survival,
and as to whom we would be very reluctant to conduct research, in
the sense of nonbeneficial research -- research that is not intended
to help them, because of the fear that that would interfere with
any ability to, in fact, live, although they are called viable.

There are other concepts which relate to the respect that is due
a subject, and I am not sure that viability will necessarily be the
bright line that separates those groups. It may be -- and I would
like to have the physicians on the panel comment on this -- it may
be that one of the things that we are concerned with is the subject's, in this case the fetus', ability in neurological terms to
experience pain. It might be, as I understand it, that development
occurs long prior to viability, but it is a concept which is not
that well understood as to what we mean by pain at that point, or
sensation, or anything like this, above the level of spinal reflexes.

Is this a concept which has to come into our definition? If we
are concerned in all of the regulation of experimentation with
preventing suffering and giving the attributes of dignity to human
beings, is viability going to be the dividing line, or do we have
to look to other factors?

JAFFE: I am not sure why, in your questioning, you direct it only to
physicians. I should like to turn the question around and ask you,
from your perspective and from a legal perspective, perhaps, or from
an ethical perspective, what do you regard as the proper criteria
for which these distinctions should be made?

CAPRON: My question, I think, has already suggested that I do see the
protection from suffering and the protection of individuals against
things that are inconsistent with human dignity -- that is to say,
types of research that we would not want to conduct on a living
human being -- as being two things with which we are very concerned
and which, I think, lie behind the last ten year's development of
guidelines from the government and increasing ethical discussions
such as this one.

I would suggest that, if you, as physicians, can supply the data,
then there would be a basis for discussion. The data relates to
the neurological development of the fetus. Is there a point prior
to viability at which you would say that, for purposes of sensation,
pain, and the like, we are dealing with something other than simply
a slightly differentiated mass of cells?

I am not sure that that will answer the question. I am not trying to say that, if the answer is yes, then, absolutely, we should recommend no research. But I think that this is the kind of datum other than that about viability which should enter into any drawing of guidelines.

ALFORD: As I understand the state of the art, it would be almost impossible to tell you now what the neurological development is of the fetus when we even are having some trouble measuring a newborn baby at this stage. Our machines that measure electrical activity really cannot be placed on the head of a very small fetus and give us any concept. If research continues, perhaps these can be answered for us in time. But, at this point in time, perhaps there really isn't any answer to some of those questions.

HAYS: I think it ought to be pointed out that the research we are talking about here doesn't really involve infliction of pain on the viable or nonviable fetus. The idea of doing something that would bear risk is the reason for not using the viable fetus in any kind of procedure. I don't think anyone on this panel would contemplate any experiment involving pain or grotesque or other manipulation of a fetus.

I would like, then, to perhaps bring this point up for discussion. It was raised this morning, and judging from the response of the audience, it is one that is on the minds of many individuals in the audience: that is, to what extent are these horror stories true? To what extent has the devastating and inhumane research been done on fetuses in this country? Does anyone have the answer to that? Isn't this a question that is somehow at the basis of a great deal of the problems that we are having here?

ROBBINS: The only study that I know that is related to this and that is at all systematic is one being conducted for the Commission, which will have, as I understand it, a pretty good catalogue of what is going on and what has been going on. I think the research that aroused a great deal of concern was research directed at understanding the capacity of the brain of the fetus to metabolize sugar, to use sugar as an energy source, in comparison to what happens in the older individual. This involved cannulating the neck vessels and, essentially, profusing the brain. This was done in small, previable fetuses. There would be no way that I know of to answer your question, Mr. Capron, as to whether or not that fetus, in fact, experienced pain.

This is the kind of thing that does sound like a horror story. The investigators who were involved in those experiments, with small fetuses where there is no evidence of electrical activity in the brain that has been detected, felt that the likelihood of any sensation of pain was so remote that it wasn't necessary to consider.

81

Now, the fact of the matter is, I don't think you can say that se-
curely. It is probable, but it isn't absolute.

RENÉE FOX: Might I make a comment in response to Mr. Capron's question.
This may be taking liberties with the preoccupations of the physicians on the platform, but --

ROBBINS: Well, you just go right ahead and take those liberties.

FOX: But I sense that they are concerned to better understand what it
is that they are working with in various stages of development of
the fetus.
      The words that we have are inadequate. But the incipient or
potential personhood of this developing creature, the actual personhood of this individual in becoming, and many things that are
paradoxically not quite so biological as the question you, as a non-
biologist, have asked, led me to muse a bit about whether, in the
end, even if we do have all the biological information we ideally
would need, if your question could be answered. Would that be adequate to allow us to grapple better than we are at the moment with
the question of this continuum of life that the fetus represents,
and to determine at what point personhood asserts itself?
      I think the factors there are not purely biological, although a
better biological understanding can help us with some dimensions of
that problem. Lawyers and sociologists and people who are non-
biological are permitted more freely to use the kinds of words that
I am using than the physicians on this platform. But I am assuming
that that is what they are really concerned about, although they
are using biomedical language to cover it.

ALFORD: We think patients are all persons.

WILLIAM CURRAN: I am from Harvard University and, like Franz Ingelfinger,
I come from Massachusetts. We have some rather serious problems
related directly to this area.
      I am not really sure that any of you has discussed consent. In
many of these cases, the concept of consent is involved. It is also
involved because of the fact that it is said that the Supreme Court,
in those decisions that Renée Fox mentioned, indicates that the
fetus, prior to viability, is not a person.
      Those two things are connected. That is, the issue of consent is
raised, not on research that is beneficial, which Dr. Brown discussed,
but in research that is said not to be directly beneficial to the
fetus. Can the mother consent for such research? If she cannot,
who can? If we need this research, what kind of institutional
determination can we suggest for providing that protection?
      Secondly, if we accept the idea that the Supreme Court indicated
that, for the purpose of protection in relation to abortion, the
fetus is not a person prior to viability, again, what are we talking
about?

82

How do we protect it? What identification do we give it? Much of the fear is that it is neither protectable nor, perhaps, even studyable.

Lastly, again, as the case in Massachusetts in which we now have had a homocide finding by a jury, we have the relationship between this subject and abortions. The statute passed in Massachusetts has two different areas of barring of fetal research, not only in regard to research involving the fetus in utero, but in the use of tissue on which at least one of you indicated you thought there were no ethical issues.

This statute bars research on a fetus for which there is a planned abortion. The position of the group that supported that did so on the basis of saying the mother, in such a situation, does not have the interest of the fetus as her main concern, and, therefore, her consent alone is not adequate. This is quite, you see, contrary to the point you made that the mother who, perhaps, is going to have an abortion and says, "Well, certainly, there should be some use here. I should be able to consent to procedures, even, perhaps, damaging procedures, because after all I am going to have an abortion anyway." Those who advocated this statute said that is quite improper, that there should be someone to protect that fetus because of the fact that there is a planned abortion.

Secondly, in it being a planned abortion, and in the other category of the use of tissues, it is alleged, again by this group, that encouragement of research in these areas will also encourage abortions. The statute bars contact with the woman prior to the time that she is going to have an abortion offering her, for example, free medical services in a particular institution as long as she gives them the fetus for purposes of research.

It seems to me that this means that we are intertwining here issues of consent, issues of who protects both the viable and the nonviable fetus, and that we clearly need, according to the research you have indicated, to be concerned with the nonviable as well as the viable fetus and these interrelated questions of abortion. It seems to me that the case of Dr. Edelin certainly raises the question. It is now, certainly, a matter of very grave concern to him whether or not, when a physician has full and proper consent from the woman for an abortion, he is doing a perfectly legal abortion. And yet, depending on what happens to the fetus, depending on what happens to his care of the fetus outside the womb, there may be an additional, completely independent responsibility for which even a homocide may lie.

One of you spoke of the physician to the fetus. I am not sure whether you meant a pediatrician or an obstetrician or someone new. It is certainly not terribly clear that the physician who cares for the woman is not primarily concerned with the woman. Perhaps it is concern with the fetus when, as you say, the research or the therapy is related to saving that fetus. But if we divorce it from this, if we put it in the category of research, it seems to me that these issues of consent, these issues of protection, have not really been adequately discussed.

JAFFE: The issue of informed consent in pregnancy is an extremely complex one, and one to which I don't feel that I should address myself in toto; for that, we do need the contributions of people other than physicians. I think, at least on a national scale, that whether or not an abortion is permissable has been decided in the courts. It is extremely important that the individual performing research on the fetus be in no way involved in the decision for an abortion on that fetus. These two should be divorced so that there are no implications that the investigator, in any way, influenced the permission or nonpermission for an abortion to be performed. I do think, however, if an abortion has been an accomplished fact, that as a physician I would much prefer some use being made of that aborted material than no use being made of it.

BATTAGLIA: I would like to begin by assuming that we are talking about a living organism, whether it is an abortus or fetus, and not living material from a dead organism. So, I come back to the biologic state that --

ROBBINS: Unfortunately, however, this luxury is not totally allowed to you by what is happening.

BATTAGLIA: Well, if I might pursue this for just a minute. I am missing how it is not allowed. But if we take the example in which it is a spontaneous abortion, and the abortus happens to be viable, whatever term we should use for it, then we would have an example in which I don't think we would have any confusion about the fact that life support systems, described by Dr. Brown, should be applied by some physician.
    So part of the confusion that is coming in is, was it an elective or a spontaneous abortion, and who is giving consent? In my talk, I was using the distinction of viability to use guidelines beyond which it is unequivocal that you would treat that living organism as a newborn infant. I wasn't using the definition of viability to say, "If it is previable and living, anything goes," by any means, and I did not use that discussion in what research I thought was appropriate.

ROBBINS: Does that even remotely answer anything, Dr. Curran?

ALFORD: He asked a simple question: Is there a new breed of cat being developed? Yes, there is a thing called perinatology that we are hoping to create. Right now it comes off the pediatric base probably more than the obstetrical base, because of our working with newborn babies in the past. This is a very, very new field. It has not been defined as to its criteria, but I can assure you that most people in

84

this area feel very strongly that the fetus is, indeed, a patient. The definition of life is something entirely different than that.

The second thing that you alluded to was that the Edelin case was in some way connected to the research. I was unaware that that was the issue. I believe the issue in this case was manslaughter, and it did not involve the research aspect, which is a second case entirely on robbing the grave in 1880 law.

CURRAN: I was referring to the others.

ALBERT MORACZEWSKI: My remarks were already anticipated in part by Professor Curran, so I won't repeat them except to pick up one point and amplify a little bit. In mentioning the fact that the Supreme Court has decided that the fetus up to a certain stage is not a person, I think a distinction here might be helpful: that is, the difference between a legal person and an ontological or ethical person.

I think there is part of a larger distinction between ethical concerns and legal concerns, and these two keep intertwining even though they are different. I think in our analysis of personhood, which is critical in the notion of fetus, if this double concept would be clarified it might help in our discussions.

Finally, who is going to give consent for and rightfully give consent for the fetus in this type of research? I would propose and I would support the idea, at least at this point, that it is an analogous situation to an infant. Who can give consent for an infant when the procedure is not going to be of benefit to that child, but rather to the class or to society at large? The same principle that is applicable there, I feel, should be applicable to fetal research.

ROBBINS: You mean you are going to answer one insoluble problem with another.

BARBARA SYSKA: I am from Maryland Right to Life, and I want to raise an ethical problem concerning the mother of the fetus. Suppose she wants to let this fetus be used for experimental purposes, and she agrees to an abortion. According to the Nuremberg Code, Item 9, which we usually use for adult experimental subjects, we are always subject to withdrawal from the experiment, whatever is the reason, whether the consent was not really informed or whether something changed.

Between the time something was done to the fetus and the abortion, there is a time lag that gives an opportunity for the woman to change her mind and, according to what we usually say, the subject has the right to withdraw from the experiment. We know so little about fetuses that we cannot assume that whatever the relation is, there is a high risk of either physical or mental disability if that fetus would be allowed to live.

Supposing the mother changes her mind, and she has a baby somehow not normal completely, either physically or mentally, someone
who can live for seventy or eighty years? Of course, there is a
legal problem of who would take care of that abnormal person, and
also who will be responsible for the damage done. But I am coming
back to the ethical problem. That woman has the right to change
her mind, but once she changes her mind and she doesn't want to have
an abortion any longer, she doesn't present that fetus for further
research. She has the problem right now of normal life for that
baby or the death of the baby.

Now, any doctor would say in that case she should really have an
abortion. Suppose she changes her mind once more? We know that
about 10 percent of the women have a very psychological sequel to
the abortion, and that one group at high risk are those who have
abortions for medical reasons. This would be a woman under high
risk. So if we allow a woman to agree to any research so that she
will have an abortion afterwards, we are taking away one of the
rights, the right to withdraw from the experiment, because she
either has an impossible choice, or --

ROBBINS: I think the message has gotten through very clearly to the
panel.

JAFFE: I think this is a very difficult question, one that the Peel
Commission has already dealt with in Great Britain, and one that I
suspect the current Commission in the United States is also dealing
with. What do we do in the event that a woman changes her mind
regarding an abortion?

The Peel Report states that, because of this concern, no investigation can be done in anticipation of an abortion. Therefore, only
investigation is permitted once the abortion has been accomplished.
This raises problems vis-à-vis very important areas that need to be
tackled prior to delivery, but it is one solution to that ethical
dilemma.

JACK HUGHES: I am a physician and currently connected with the Yale
University School of Medicine. My question is directed to you,
Dr. Robbins.

So far we have had a parade of speakers, the overwhelming majority
of whom have been fairly highly placed in the biomedical establishment, if you will. Not surprisingly, their comments have all been
in defense of the conduct of the current biomedical research. It
disturbs me somewhat that the challenges have to come from the floor.
This meeting was advertised as a forum, and not as a defense of biomedical research as it is presently conducted. Wouldn't it be
possible to have some of the adversaries on the podium to give presentations along with the people who are defending the current
biomedical research?

ROBBINS: Yes, indeed. Actually, as a matter of fact, that was our original intent. It didn't work out quite that way.

GEORGE HILL: I am what is called an interested citizen.

ROBBINS: We welcome you, sir.

HILL: Thank you very much. I feel I have been somewhat lucky to be able to sit here in this discussion. It seems to me that one of the issues that has been avoided from the beginning concerns the fluid, placenta, and the tissues of a fetus whether viable or not. Is it true that a new industry is being developed around them because of their immense importance in chemical and biological developments for pharmaceuticals?

My second question is: Why not give the woman who has an abortion or has a nonviable fetus the property rights to that? Those property rights should be paid for by the hospital or by those pharmaceutical houses that are going to use the fetus for experimental purposes. This would solve the very interesting problem as to whether the fetus belongs to the woman and should be paid for by those who exploit it for whatever purposes, including patent rights and whatever.

I introduce these difficulties to show that even the physicians and the theologians are not quite prepared to grasp the very important ingredient of our society -- private property. Is a fetus private property? Is it salable? Under what conditions? Perhaps, the Supreme Court will discuss that. I might say that one of the important ingredients in solving this problem is to place either a physician or a scientist on the next vacancy of the Supreme Court. That would certainly solve the situation.

ROBBINS: I am afraid that might really foul things up.

JAFFE: I could very briefly address the first part of your question; I don't think I have the legal or ethicist background to discuss the second. There are valid uses to be made of placentas, not just from aborted fetuses, but from all placentas, including those from women in term after a living baby is delivered. Hormones, blood clotting factors, and other valuable material for medical practice can be derived from them. And, indeed, there have been commercial uses made of these, just as there are commercial sales of antibiotics. Personally, I don't feel that this is inappropriate.

ROBBINS: As far as I know, except for the fact that some cells derived from fetal tissue have been established in tissue culture and maintained to grow viruses for vaccine purposes, fetal tissues, in themselves, have never had a market.

FOX: If I could make one other comment. In listening even to the most modest and the least arrogant of us, I think we keep saying that we can answer only this part of a question, or that it lies outside of our competence. All of us are disclaiming to have the range of competencies, even when we are put together, that would make us collectively the ultimate arbiters of the questions that are being posed in this Forum.

I come back to the Supreme Court, because sociologically speaking this is the body in our land that, in a nation under laws rather than under men, normally would be considered to be the supreme group to speak for the collectivity on issues that are at once legally and morally relevant. Yet a number of the comments we have made today suggest -- and this is not out of disrespect to the Supreme Court of our land -- that we are into an area where we can't separate out a constellation of issues. If that case of Roe vs. Wade should have to be tried again and go all the way up to the top of the court system and our judges would have to sit again on those considerations, the next decision, for example, would have as many loopholes, would have as many questions about personhood and when it begins.

I suppose a social scientist should be able to give the magical answer to this. But do we have current organizations and mechanisms available to us in our society for the arbitration of complex questions of this kind -- I refer not to just special groups, but to all of us -- and adequate to deal with these questions at hand? I think we are suggesting that maybe not. I don't know whether this is the group to get involved in making a new social invention, but I am sort of confronted with that problem.

JOSEPH BELLANTI: I am a physician and a professor at Georgetown University, and I would like to say a word in behalf of fetal research. As a Catholic and as a professor at a Catholic institution, I can handle both the problem of fetal research as well as the convictions of my religion. Any discussion of fetal research inextricably is wound and tied together with the problem of abortion. I think we have to separate those two issues. Clearly, one's belief about abortion is one thing, and one's belief about fetal research is another.

I am a proponent of fetal research provided that it preserves the dignity and the worth of humans. I have participated in fetal research within the bounds of my convictions. I have obtained phymic tissue from fetuses and reconstituted children suffering from immune deficiency. In a sense, we have saved the lives of others. The problems related to abortion are separate. In confusing the two, I think we do the cause of fetal research a disservice. I would just like to make that point very clear.

KENNETH GOETZ: I am Director of Experimental Medicine at St. Luke's Hospital, Kansas City. Although I am a licensed physician, I consider myself, primarily, a scientific biologist. I am also a former

88

fetus. I would agree in some cases that abortion and fetal research can be separated. However, if the fetal research implies the death of the fetus, I think that you are talking about the same thing.

Now, I have struggled with this question for several years and the thing that bothers me mostly, as a biologist, is when I look at it statistically. I look at each of us here having a life cycle, which starts from the day of conception with forty-six specific chromosomes that make us unique in that sense. It seems to me that, therefore, the bright line we talked about a short time ago seems to be very out of focus and very hazy. What is the difference between one week and the next in utero? I confess that I cannot see it. When a fetus is something like six weeks old, the statistical probability of its being born, unless we as medical scientists do something about it, is perhaps 90 percent. The obstetricians and embryologists can correct me on that. The problem we have to think about is that, statistically, you are going to chop off a life cycle very early; perhaps euthanasia, at the other end of the cycle, in some ways would be less unpalatable.

MURIEL NELLIS: I am a special consultant to the United Methodist General Welfare Board, specifically the Office of Drugs and Alcohol, with particular emphasis, in recent years, on women and health.

There has been reference to the physician to the fetus, and Dr. Brown was pleased to note in her opening remarks that finally researchers, pediatricians, and obstetricians seem to be coming together in common cause. I think that, in order to bring that full cycle, we ought to go back to square one. I have heard no comment or concern here, nor any sense of assumed responsibility on the part of any of those disciplines, with respect to: the carrier of the fetus and maternal health, such regulatory agencies' behavior as the FDA in regard to oral contraceptives and additional hormones into the prescriptions for women, the myriad of those hormones in our food chain, or the possible consequences of taking a cumulative look by way of research rather than continuing on this path of isolated individual examination of tolerance levels of one drug or another. The possibility that fetuses and women are contaminated with government approval is an abhorrent notion, but nonetheless, it seems to me, a very real possibility right now. As you are concerned with the health of women and the ultimate health of their progeny, perhaps one ought to start examining what we are doing or not doing by way of new levels of tolerance level management and research with respect to the hormones that we are ingesting and being prescribed, as well as Red Dye 2 and all of those things either taken sequentially or simultaneously.

I will pose one question. Does anyone here know of a single piece of basic research whose purpose is intended to determine, in addition to cattle, whether in women there are residues after any period of time of ingestion either through the food chain or through prescriptions of any of these known carcinogenic chemicals?

JAFFE: That type of investigation, of course, would be proscribed at present in the pregnant woman. In the nonpregnant individual there are attempts made to assess how much of a given hormone is cleared of the body, how much of it is metabolized and broken down to inactive hormones, and how much of it is retained.

You are posing a very big problem, which, unfortunately, can only be gotten at a piece at a time. Yes, there are investigations designed to look at how hormones work, what they may be doing that is beneficial, and what they may be doing that is harmful. There is no big sweeping study, which would utilize millions and millions of dollars, that I am aware of to attack the whole problem at once.

ROBBINS: I might say that you are proposing an extraordinarily difficult experimental problem.

DORIS HAIRE: First of all, I would like to say that diethylstilbestrol is still being administered to women who choose not to breast-feed. I was in a hospital not too long ago where I saw it being used.

My major concern, today, is that so much has been expounded over the condition of the fetus that will be destroyed. I would like to bring up the fact that virtually none of the drugs presently given to pregnant, parturient women have ever been established as safe in regard to their long-term effects on the child. We have one in every thirty-three children today being diagnosed as retarded, and one in every seventeen as having some form of significant learning dysfunction. None of these drugs presently being used, and presently being used in research, have ever been proven safe for the unborn child. I think we are missing the boat.

THE CHILD

William C. Smith
Leon Eisenberg
Charles R. Halpern

WILLIAM SMITH

There hasn't been much controversy in these proceedings so far, and I
don't think there has been very much serious discussion of ethical
issues involved in medical research. The last panel was in total agreement about everything that they were willing to discuss or give answers
to. There was no reluctance at all this morning to keeping the federal
government out of the research business. There has been a lot of
reluctance this afternoon, so far, to discuss informed consent and
ethical issues and the other things that I think this Forum is supposed
to be about.

What we have tried to do is put together the following case that we
hope will change the level of discussion and open up some debate.

Hypothetical Case

Haym's Syndrome is a disease of the joints that begins in early
childhood and becomes progressively more debilitating through early
adulthood, severely impairing joint function in about half the cases.
The death rate among Haym's Syndrome victims is about 10 percent
before age eighteen, increasing throughout adulthood to about 40 percent by age forty.

All groups within the American population are at equal risk for
this disease.

There is a conventional treatment that may bring symptom relief,
but there is no known cure.

Several competent investigators concluded after six months of animal studies that a new drug, NAS-18, if administered continuously in high dosages could well arrest the progress of the disease.

Their animal trials, however, have also indicated several discomforting although not serious side effects, including diarrhea and insomnia.

The investigators decided on a two-year trial at their Haym's Syndrome Clinic at University Hospital. In their NIH grant application the trial was stated to have the dual purpose of measuring the toxicity and the beneficial effects of NAS-18 and weighing them against each other.

Forty potential subjects were selected. Thirty were outpatients at the Haym's Syndrome Clinic. Of these thirty, ten were children ranging in age from five to seventeen.

One of the investigators was the staff physician at the local juvenile training school. Ten adolescents age ten to fifteen at the school had Haym's Syndrome and were therefore selected as the remaining subjects.

At their next clinic visit, each of the thirty outpatients -- twenty adults and a parent of each of the ten child subjects -- was asked to participate in the research project. One of the investigators carefully explained the following to each person:

-- That NAS-18 was a new drug that had shown promising results in previous tests. It might possibly be a major breakthrough in the campaign against Haym's Syndrome, and it might lessen the subject's pain. No one, however, could be sure of this until further research was undertaken.
-- That the procedure simply involved taking pills on a regular basis and that their progress would be carefully monitored.
-- That previous research had indicated some chance of developing the known side effects described earlier but that there could be other, unknown side effects.

The patients and the parents of the child subjects were then given a chance to ask questions and asked to sign the standard consent form used by University Hospital. [That form follows the statement of the case.]

Parental consent was obtained for all but three of the ten training school subjects whose parents could not be located. The school's chief administrator's consent also was obtained. The subjects then met as a group with the investigator and were told that they were being asked to participate in a drug test that had been approved by the administrator. They were given the same information as the clinic patients, but they were not asked to sign a consent form. They were told that they could withdraw from the experiment at any time.

The research proceeded according to design. Half the adults and half the children were given NAS-18, the other half a placebo. Dosages for all subjects were increased periodically during the first year of the research.

Many of the subjects seemed to benefit substantially from the administration of NAS-18 -- especially the children whose disease had not progressed to its most debilitating stages. All subjects on NAS-18 experienced less pain.

However, at a dosage where NAS-18 appeared to slow the progress of the disease, five subjects developed peripheral neuropathy, three so severe they had trouble walking. The investigators took all five subjects off NAS-18 and reduced the dosage administered to the other fifteen.

Neither the remaining fifteen NAS-18 subjects nor the twenty control subjects were informed of the neuropathy. Four months later five more subjects developed peripheral neuropathy. They then were taken off the drug.

Near the end of the trial, many of the subjects whose symptoms had been most relieved told the investigators they wanted to continue NAS-18 treatments. Expecting an affirmative response, they were surprised and disappointed when told that further trials were necessary before NAS-18 could be approved as accepted treatment for Haym's Syndrome and that they could not continue on the drug after the end of the two-year trial.

At the conclusion of the experiment, all patients were taken off NAS-18, told that further research would be undertaken but not at University Hospital, and thanked for their cooperation and help in finding what appeared to be a promising therapy for Haym's Syndrome.

Six patients who continued to show abnormal nerve conduction and signs of peripheral neuropathy continued their visits to the clinic.

We have chosen this hypothetical case because it raises serious and debatable issues. This experiment should never have been approved by the University's Research Review Committee or funded by the National Institutes of Health. The researchers gave children a drug that was never before tested on humans. There was no need for this, and no justification. Children should not have been used until the toxicity of NAS-18 had first been tested on adults, especially since the experiment could, at best, have benefited the subjects only temporarily. Even captive children were used, and used purely for the convenience of the investigators. Institutionalized children should not have been placed at risk when other subjects were available.

Three children were used without the consent of even their parents. No child, at least one of whose natural or adoptive parents were not available to give informed consent, should be the subject of a nontherapeutic experiment. None of the children were themselves asked to consent. I submit that no child over seven should be placed at risk in a nontherapeutic experiment without his or her approval.

UNIVERSITY HOSPITAL

Program of Clinical Investigation

PATIENT'S CONSENT

I _____, understand that the
physicians at University Hospital are engaged in diagnosis and
treatment of diseases, research on the nature of diseases and
investigation of methods of diagnosis and treatment. I have
been informed of the nature of the program of clinical investigation and procedures that is/are briefly described as:

ADMINISTRATION OF NAS-18 FOR HAYM'S SYNDROME

My physician has explained to me the procedures to be followed,
identifying those that are experimental. He has also described
the possible discomforts and risks as well as the benefits to be
expected. I have been informed concerning the availability of
appropriate alternative procedures that might be advantageous
for me.
   I have had the opportunity to ask questions concerning the
   procedures. I further understand that I am free to withdraw
   my consent and discontinue participation in the study at any
   time.
   I hereby voluntarily consent to participate in this study
   and voluntarily consent that treatment and diagnostic procedures as described above may be performed on me.

_____   _____
(Signature of patient or legal guardian)   (Date)

_____
(Witness) Cannot be the Physician

_____
NOTE: If there is anything that you do not understand about
       this explanation, ask the doctor for further information.
_____

PHYSICIAN'S STATEMENT

I have offered an opportunity for further explanation of this
procedure to the individual whose signature appears above.

                    _____
                          (Signature)

94

In this experiment both children and adults were misused. True informed consent requires complete disclosure. The University Hospital investigators failed to disclose that a major goal of the experiment was to determine the toxicity of NAS-18. They failed to disclose that the drug had never before been tried on humans. They did not tell the subjects that an alternative treatment that might relieve their symptoms was available. They failed to disclose that every subject had a fifty-fifty chance of receiving a placebo. They failed to tell the subjects that the experiment would end in two years, and that even if the subjects benefited from NAS-18, they would not be permitted to continue this drug therapy. And when neuropathy appeared in a few subjects, the researchers failed to reobtain consent in light of the new danger; they failed, in fact, even to inform the others of the most recently discovered risk.

It should be noted that the subjects used were the doctors' patients. The Hippocratic Oath states: "The health and life of my patient will be my first consideration." That Oath was broken in this case. The investigators' primary interest was not in their patients but in their research. As a result, they used patients who should not have been subjected to research, and they used them needlessly and irresponsibly. A physician who uses his patients as research subjects inevitably places himself in a conflict between his role as healer and his role as research investigator. I seriously question whether any physician should be permitted to conduct a nontherapeutic experiment on his or her own patients. Certainly a research subject's health interest should always be protected by a third party not involved in the research.

I began by stating that this case should never have been approved by the University Hospital's Research Review Committee. I do not think it would have been approved if such research review committees were properly constituted. Decisions about risks and benefits, how subjects are to be selected, and the adequacy of disclosure and consent are too important to be left to the medical research profession, persons with a vested interest in the outcome of their own and their colleagues' work.

I suggest it is time that review committees be required to open their meetings to the public. We have heard a lot of talk about openness this morning. I think it is the peer review process that needs to be opened up to public scrutiny. I suggest also that it is high time that the peer review process involve not just the peers of the researchers, but the peers of the subjects as well.

LEON EISENBERG

This panel is not one of unanimity. I would like to tell a clinical vignette to illuminate the situation.

All of you are familiar with the time when Moses arrived at the Red Sea with a multitude of the Jews chased by the armies of the pharaoh. At that point he turned to the terribly distressed group, who saw the

Red Sea ahead of them, and said that he had both good news and bad news. The good news, as he announced it, was that the Red Sea would divide in the middle so they could go through on dry land, that they would arrive on the other side just as the pharaoh's army entered, that the sea would close again, and that they would emerge victorious. There was loud cheering until a small chap at the back of the crowd said, "What is the bad news?"

"Well, the bad news is that before I can do it, we have to file an environmental impact statement."

To turn to the other side of the question, I have another story. When the Archbishop of Canterbury, the Chief Rabbi, the Pope, and the Grand Mufti were killed in a plane crash en route to an ecumenical congress on the Ethics of Medical Research, all four, as was to be expected, were admitted to Heaven without unseemly delay. They were, however, somwhat perturbed to learn that there were no privileged elites in Heaven. Each of the multitude of souls had to wait his -- or worse, *her* -- turn in the cafeteria line when meals were served. This was a bit awkward. But being men of vast and humane scholarship, they recognized the justice of the contemporary trend toward egalitarianism. After some days of rather painless acculturation to celestial life- styles, they were quite put out when a short bearded man wearing a white cap and gown elbowed his way to the front of the dinner line, demanded and was granted immediate service. Their Eminences insisted upon an explanation, only to be told -- "Shh! That's God! He likes to play doctor."

Although I have this story from a reliable source, I will not insist on its authenticity. Apocryphal as the tale may be, it represents conventional wisdom about medical behavior. There *are* doctors who enjoy playing God, perhaps even some who entered medicine precisely because they saw no other avenue to deification so readily at hand and with so little risk of being certified as lunatic. Doctors are to be found at every level of ethical sensitivity, including none at all; but I insist, so are lawyers, judges, philosophers, and theologians. What does distinguish physicians is the tradition, centuries old, to guide our behavior in clinical transactions. We have been assigned, from time before history, the agonizing task of confronting suffering and death, most often without means adequate to alter their course, but with very broad sanctions from society.

What has been, of course, is not necessarily what is best -- even if sufficient to its time, may no longer suffice. But before we en- code, legislate, and thus inevitably bureaucratize medical ethics, caution may not be inappropriate. The very informality of the tradi- tional relationship between physician and patient, for all the risk of abuse it entails, may be the talisman that permits particularized and personal solutions for matters in which ambiguities inhere. It is just possible that the social cost of erecting legal barriers against the possibility of harm may be the elimination of a far greater benefit conferred by the flexibility of general and necessarily imprecise guidelines.

These prefatory remarks are stimulated by a climate of opinion, at least in Massachusetts, which almost explicitly implies that medical researchers are mad, or at least self-serving, scientists from whom the public, as potential victim, must be protected by the benevolent inter-position of courts, theologians, and assorted humanists. I suggest that all parts of that proposition merit searching examination before being received as the revealed truth.

The current zeal for zero risk, a goal by definition unattainable when research by its nature is a venture into the unknown, threatens the very possibility of acquiring that new knowledge which might prevent present harm and permit future good. Drugs and procedures in current use, sanctioned by familiarity and lacking the label *research*, are readily assumed to be of established value when they may rest on no more than custom. Withholding them, or substituting novel items, courts public outrage. Yet controlled therapeutic trial is the principal avenue to evaluating their effectiveness. When other physicians fled Philadelphia during the epidemic of yellow fever in 1793, Benjamin Rush, dedicated to his calling, remained at his post after bundling his family off to the safety of the countryside. Messianic in his zeal for purging and blood-letting, therapeutic maneuvers based on contemporary authority, he went from home to plague-ridden home, causing more carnage than the disease itself. Good intention and willingness to undergo personal risk provided no substitute for knowledge then, nor do they now.

Health is hazard to fashion when we impose standards for therapeutic trials that demand assurances of safety and efficacy beyond those that can be offered for the best of contemporary medical practice. The current preoccupation with the dangers of research, dangers that un-questionably merit public discussion, is uncommonly set in the appro-priate context: namely, weighing on the same scale the dangers of *not* doing research. Some would have us regard the percentage of research proposals rejected by a human studies committee as a measure of its effectiveness in protecting the public interest, without independently assessing the scientific and ethical soundness of the approved or dis-approved protocols themselves. Clearly, kudos for the highest research rejection batting average imply that the proper target for the review committee is blocking human studies. To the contrary, I suggest that the systematic imposition of impediments to significant therapeutic research is itself unethical because potential benefit is being denied. This is not a call for unrestricted rights for medical researchers by invoking the suffering of mankind as justification. It is a plea to weigh the cost-benefit ratios in both directions. The decision not to do something poses as many ethical quandaries as the decision to do it. Not to act is to act.

Let us now turn to the protocol for NAS-18 and the hypothetical case that our panel has put before you. We can agree that the first trials should have been limited to adults. Nonetheless, that step would have lessened but would not have eliminated the hazard in a subsequent pedi-atric trial. There is significant residual ambiguity about probable effect when a drug is first used on an infant or a child even after exhaustive animal tests, because of interspecific differences, and after its use in the human adult, because of developmental differences. Rate of absorption, body distribution, detoxification, excretion, and end organ responsiveness differ between the infant, the child, and the adult. Beyond these promptly detectable effects is the deeply troublesome question of long-term consequences for growth and development. One need only recall the potent effect of sex hormones given during pregnancy or at birth on the organogenesis, sexual development, and subsequent behavior of the organism, when there is no longer any chemical residue of the drug.

Suffice it to say, there is a nontrivial risk whenever a drug is given for the first time to a child. Further, the more potent the drug in treating the condition at which it is directed, the greater the risk of undesired side effects. Inevitably, the more widely the drug is used, the greater the likelihood of encountering idiosyncratic responses not previously anticipated.

Even if risk in research be inevitable, inequity in exposure to risk need not be. As in the hypothetical protocol, the patients on whom research is most often done are clinic patients. In the past this has been explicitly justified on the grounds that this was the price exacted from the poor for the privilege of receiving charity care. Few would defend that position today. Yet it continues, less by plan or conspiracy than by the nature of the medical care system. Investigators are located in teaching hospitals. Teaching hospitals are a major medical resource for the poor. The poor become the patients on whom studies are done. There is no justification for putting particular segments of the population at risk unless the disease under study is itself limited to such populations. I doubt that we will find a way of distributing risk across all segments of society until we have a national health service for all citizens. Only then will it be possible to guarantee equity by distributing risk randomly, once we agree that the assumption of risk for social benefit is the responsibility to be shared by all citizens.

A second difficult question inheres in the meaning of informed consent. When risks are specifiable, when it is possible for the patient to make a rational decision, it is clearly the physician's duty to inform the patient fully. That has long been a hallmark of good medical practice and sound clinical investigation, although it has become fashionable to present it as contemporary discovery. But what does *informed* mean when what is available to the physician, let alone the patient, is not information but noise? In what sense is there a choice to be made between Treatment A and Treatment B if there is no proof that either works or that one is superior to the other? What right have I lost if I, in a national health plan, am assigned to a randomized trial without being free to express a preference when that preference can only be capricious? If there is evidence that Treatment A is better or less toxic than Treatment B, my doctor is incompetent as well as irresponsible if he does not recommend A and press it upon

me with all the force of his moral suasion. The very justification of
a randomized trial is the lack of information to permit a rational,
that is, an informed choice.

All will agree that when the patients are children their parents must
be fully informed and permitted unconstrained choice. This immediately
identifies two violations in the NAS-18 protocol: the use of a captive
population (i.e., the delinquents in a training school) and youngsters
without a responsible parent. None or few would argue that the concept
of informed consent is appropriate for the infant or the very young
child. But some, like Mr. Smith, insist upon its applicability, even
after parents have exercised their role, for the child seven years of
age or older. I fail to understand how a child with an illness threat-
ening life or limb can "decide" whether to be treated, or when to choose
the standard treatment or the experimental one. Should we let children
decide whether they want to take an immunosuppressive drug for leukemia,
or insulin and diet for diabetes? In what real way is it meaningful to
propose that a child should elect whether or not to enter a clinical
trial when the immediate aspects of the procedure -- discomfort, restriction, awesomeness and the like -- can be expected to outweigh his or her
ability to reckon with the long-term consequences of the illness? We
are being asked to ratify a legal formalism that fails to correspond
with the realities of cognitive and affective development.

Some groups and individuals, in the name of children's rights, would
go further. They would deny parents the authority to consent to therapeutic trials for their children without the interposition of a court-
appointed guardian to represent the child's interests. It is true that
there are parents who, burdened by a handicapped or difficult child,
might welcome the chance to be rid of him. Indeed, once in my career,
a father and a mother volunteered their child for "any experiment you
suggest" even though none had been proposed to them. But such parents
are rare. Further, it should be an ethical imperative for clinical
investigators and research review committees to protect children from
harm from whatever source. The routine imposition of the court between
parent and child would threaten the family trust and integrity that
government should preserve. I remain to be convinced that courts will
be wiser, on average, than parents and pediatricians. I know that they
will be slower; children's rights do not keep well.

I see no justification for the use of a "placebo" in the protocol
rather than the "conventional treatment" as a basis for comparison,
since we are told that conventional treatment brings symptom relief.
Further, it was unethical to withhold information on the unexpected
toxic neuropathy. But I do not accept Mr. Smith's proposition that
"researchers...not use as subjects persons with whom they have established a doctor-patient relationship." Clinical investigators are
likely to be just those physicians most knowledgeable about the disease
under study, the ones with a large group of patients they are caring for
and whose care they seek to improve. Shall investigation be restricted
to physicians with limited experience and few patients? The altogether
remarkable progress in the development of anti-leukemic agents for

children with leukemia was the work of precisely those clinicians with the greatest experience in the treatment of leukemic children, and the subjects of the therapeutic trials were those doctors' patients.

Knowledge and involvement are the preconditions for ethical judgments. Ignorance may assure disinterest; it also guarantees misfortune.

CHARLES HALPERN

Roughly speaking, ten of the last twelve speakers at this microphone have come to the subject of human experimentation via the laboratories and clinical research, including Leon Eisenberg. I have come to the problem of human experimentation, particularly with children, from a quite different direction, and I think that direction is relevant to my response to the Haym's Syndrome case that we presented and to the proceedings thus far.

I came to the practice of human experimentation in the Partlow State School for the Mentally Retarded in Tuscaloosa, Alabama. This was not a field in which I had any training or specialization, and what I found in the Partlow State School, quite apart from the human experimentation issues, was a shock and an education in itself.

More shocking still, however, was my discovery that some of the worst abuses of mentally retarded children were under the direct supervision of Ph.D.'s and M.D.'s, were undertaken in the name of scientific research, and were funded by the Department of Health, Education, and Welfare. When I investigated this practice I discovered what I am sure most of you know: that our institutions for the mentally retarded historically have been a free fire zone for biomedical researchers. It is not in Alabama alone that you find these kinds of situations. One need only to go to an institution like Willowbrook, in New York, to see not only the practice of eighteenth-century medicine, but also highly sophisticated biomedical research undertaken on these children.

What has emerged in the past few years is attention to problems of human experimentation from those who do not approach the problem from the angle and perspective of the biomedical researcher. Particularly lawyers and social scientists are showing a healthy interest in human experimentation in general, and in particular to those experiments that are undertaken on research subject populations who are least able to care for themselves: the mentally impaired, children, prisoners, and other people who are involuntarily confined and, for that reason, less able to negotiate with experimenters in their own interests. It is, I think, significant that on this panel we have two attorneys, William Smith and myself, who are actively involved in advocacy undertakings on behalf of these disadvantaged populations. And on tomorrow's program Alvin Bronstein will discuss the situation from the prisoners' perspective -- a group with which he has been actively involved. I think it is one of the outstanding features of this Forum that such advocates who share the perspective of subjects in the experimental process have been included on the program.

100

Let me make briefly three points about the Haym's Syndrome case
that you have been presented with, and then some more general observations based on the case and on this morning's discussion of human experimentation in general.

First, with regard to the case: I concur in Bill Smith's judgment
that the consent obtained, whether from children or adults, was grossly
inadequate. There was a failure to give adequate information on which
decisions could be made. Further, there was really a failure to obtain
the consent of the children involved in the process. According to the
facts that were set out in the description, some of these children were
as old as seventeen years. That they could adequately understand as
well as their parents or their guardian the nature of the risks they
were being asked to assume, is I think, self-evident.

A second question to emerge from this case study is the one of
where the human use committee or the peer review committee was throughout all these proceedings. The protocol in itself, as it is very
briefly sketched in, has obvious failings. In particular a peer review
committee should look closely at the procedure by which informed consent is to be obtained. Clearly, there was no such inquiry here.
Further, the peer review committee has a continuing obligation to monitor the experimental process as it moves forward. Clearly, there was
no continuing monitoring in this case, or the neuropathology that
emerged in the course of the trial would have necessitated a basic
reevaluation of the entire research design.

The third point to be made about this study is its total failure
to deal with the special problems of institutionalized children and
children without parents. Instead of simply side-stepping a consent
procedure, efforts should have been made to bolster the capacity of
these children to understand the procedure and to give an adequate
consent. If we are dealing with children in their late teens, surely
by the appointment of some sort of independent specialist or the like
it would have been possible to assure their actual consent.

Most egregiously in this experimental description is the fact that
the investigators were willing to accept the consent of a superinten-
dent to an institution, as if that were the consent of children
resident in that institution. I think the history of abuses of institutionalized children and the failures of such superintendents to
adequately safeguard their interests clearly establish that a consent
of that kind if grossly inadequate. The Haym's case, in the dimensions
that I have tried to highlight, is particularly distressing because the
HEW Regulations that were issued in August of 1974, allegedly with the
intention of safeguarding less competent populations, institutionalize
and continue some of the abuses reflected in the case.

First, they would carry the peer review committee over into institutions for the mentally ill and mentally retarded where the risks of
overreaching by the investigator are even greater. Peer review may
make sense if we are dealing with an academic community. If we are
dealing with an isolated mental hospital somewhere in upstate New York,

where there is no group of scientific peers closely observing the process, it is a totally inadequate safeguard.

Second, the HEW Regulations would permit superintendents of institutions for the mentally retarded to give their consent instead of the consent of the mentally incompetent residents in those institutions -- an invitation, I suggest, to abuse of the kind we all have a common interest in avoiding.

Finally, in the HEW Regulations, because they do not require case-by-case individualized review of the adequacy of consent, there is no assurance that adequate information on which to make an intelligent judgment will be provided to potential research subjects.

In my remaining time, let me make a few general points, triggered by this morning's discussions as well as this particular study. Dr. Moore cautioned us to avoid "the folly of abstract and general formulation" in an effort to control the process of biomedical research. It may be folly to be too precise about general formulations, but to provide explicit and reasonably understandable guidelines for researchers is vitally important. This is, to a lawyer, self-evident. What we are dealing with, when we deal with a legal process, is a set of rules and a set of procedures to assure that those rules are reliably enforced. The enterprise of human experimentation should be viewed as one that takes place within a framework of law, of rules, and one in which procedures are provided to assure that those rules are equitably enforced. The rules need not be so precise as to tie the hands of experimenters; but they can be and must be sufficiently precise to provide a framework in which the experimental process takes place. For example, it is a reasonably well-understood and properly understood rule that informed consent be provided by a subject to research, with a few limited exceptions. This is a rule that is important in itself and that should be backed by adequate procedures to assure that it is not disregarded.

A second observation: self-policing within the scientific community has not been good enough, particularly where we are dealing with human subjects who are disadvantaged by incapacitation for reasons of mental deficiency or people who are incarcerated. There have been gross abuses in the past in our institutions for the mentally retarded, in other juvenile institutions, in prisons, and in mental hospitals. It is insufficient to say that the scientific community has regulated itself and should be permitted to continue to regulate itself. I am saying no more than the obvious proposition that scientists doing research in such institutions are not above the law. If a treating physician is prohibited from using certain kinds of treatment modalities, such as, for example, electric shock with large cattle prods in order to keep patients quiet, it is no more acceptable to use such interventions and strategies if the purpose is allegedly a research purpose.

A third point I have mentioned briefly and would like to state again, is that peer review is not translatable from the university context into institutional settings; and the HEW Regulations that are written as if it were commit a serious error.

Finally, let me make two points about the present state of development of public regulation of the process of human experimentation.

We are at a point at which regulation of human experimentation should be approached from an experimental perspective. When we develop new mechanisms or translate old mechanisms from one set to another, we should do it with an experimental cast of mind, and we should structure those undertakings in a fashion that is going to give us useable data. Perhaps the most shocking thing to lay people is how little is known about what experimentation is going on, where, and under what safeguards.

When I was in Michigan recently I discovered to my surprise, for example, that the Commissioner of Mental Health did not know which mental institutions in his state had experimentation going on, or what the nature and character of such experimentation might be. It is important that we begin gathering data on what research with children, and with others, is going on now, and try to develop some ways of learning what the consequences on the experimental process would be of interposing various kinds of limitations and controls on experimentation. What, for example, would be the consequence on the development of new knowledge if we were simply to say that there will be no more experimentation in institutions for the mentally retarded? I don't think anyone can even speculate reliably on that subject.

Finally, in approaching the problem of imposing controls on human experimentation, I would like to come back to a point that was discussed briefly and inconclusively this morning: the manner in which decisions can be institutionalized. This is a point that Renée Fox touched on in her introduction. I think it is quite true that existing decision-making institutions are inadequate for resolving the difficult questions posed by human experimentation. It is too late in the game to go back to a process that relies on the principal investigator to make all and every ethical judgment that arises in the context of his experimental design. Equally clear, I think, and emerging with greater clarity, is that the courts are very blunt and inadequate instruments for making these kinds of judgments. A collaborative effort on the part of the research community and other interested persons, including representatives of subject populations, is urgently needed to develop new kinds of institutional arrangements for making these kinds of decisions. In practical terms, new careers could be created that would facilitate these kinds of decisions. Should not social workers, for example, interest themselves in the process by which informed consent is obtained and assured? Shouldn't lawyers be educated in the problems relevant to experimentation so that they can advise subjects, so that they can advise experimenters, so that they can advise those institutions that house experimental programs?

A theme that was sounded this morning was that the matter should be left to scientists. I think it is already too late for that resolution. What is needed is a constructive collaboration between research scientists and others and an explicit recognition that the problems of human experimentation have not only medical and scientific dimensions, but also ethical dimensions, legal dimensions, and political dimensions.

DON JONES: I am a professor of medicine at Wayne State University, Detroit. I think this has been a very useful panel so far, because it has hit on some problems that we have dealt with, and I would just like to give our viewpoint.

I am chairman of our Ethics Committee. One of the main things that we have had trouble with, and Mr. Halpern has brought out, is the fact that we need somebody to turn to for help with these decisions; although we have theologians from several faiths, laymen on the committee as well as scientists, we have great trouble with these, as you can imagine. I am in full agreement with both Dr. Fox and Mr. Halpern that some kind of forum be developed so people can turn to this area for help.

The problem of monitoring becomes very important in a university of limited resources. It is hard enough to get enough people to be on the committee and to be loyal to it, let alone to act as policemen, too. So I am bringing up that as a practical issue.

As to public openness, I think most committees really trying to do their jobs do have public forums. One of our most lively discussions had not to do with patients but with chimpanzees, as a matter of fact, and we had an open forum with the Humane Society on that and finally solved it. But it reminds me a little bit of a panel here at the National Academy on alcoholism in which one of the doctors was describing how he had trained his chimpanzees to speak, and the question of informed consent immediately came up for the chimpanzees.

I hope that we will address ourselves to the idea of getting some kind of a national panel. The only area we can turn to at the present time is the Institutional Relations Branch of DHEW, and they have been very helpful and very useful, but I wonder if they are the ones to make these decisions for us.

KARL COHEN: I am in the Department of Philosophy at the University of Michigan.

Let me say first, with respect to the case that was presented in hypothetical form for us, that it is not really very helpful, because I would suggest that any self-respecting human subject review committee would bounce it with very little attention, and it calls for no very careful inspection to give that result. But there are some difficult questions raised in the course of the discussion of it. One of these I would like to direct to Mr. Halpern, whose spirit I largely, although not wholly, share, and that concerns the kind of consent one must seek from youngsters who are in a position to give consent and yet are technically minors. With you I am outraged in the instant case that persons of teenage and above are not asked for their consent in an experiment of this sort.

With Professor Eisenberg I understand that there are circumstances in which one cannot oblige consent of minors of middling age, and I would ask you, Mr. Halpern, and you, Dr. Eisenberg, if you could help us in this inquiry into the problem of consent concerning youngsters, help us to formulate principles according to which consent should be obligatory, encouraged, almost obligatory, and the like. Clearly the rule of seventeen years old is absurd. I think most in the hall will agree with that. But there may be some chronological rule that is helpful, or there may be some other principles that are helpful in this respect. It seems to me that it is just in this sphere that a forum of this kind might make some real progress.

EISENBERG: Well, I think that you and I would agree that at seventeen one is as adult in all likelihood as one is going to be. At seven, one is likely to have a long distance to go. And there must be some point in between at which informed consent may begin to be meaningful and not before. I guess the difficulty in answering the problem deals with one of the serious issues that we have before us. Is there to be trust in the relationship between the hospital, the institution, the physicians, and the public, and those monitoring the care? Or is there no trust, and therefore must everything be spelled out? If one could write a set of regulations that agreed that one would look at each instance, at the nature of the child, the child's understanding, and the appropriateness of a procedure for a given age, then I am sure that Charles and I would have no difficulty agreeing that it is reasonable for Smith but not for Jones. It is difficult for me to imagine how one writes that into a codebook without so restricting freedom that you end up getting informed consent from someone at seventeen who is really incompetent, and then failing to get it from someone at twelve who might have more understanding than the seventeen-year-old.

SMITH: I just want to make a couple of comments about the informed consent of children. Obviously one has to distinguish between children of different ages. I would not apply an informed consent rule in a therapeutic situation. I would define a therapeutic situation very narrowly, however. Where the child is too young to understand -- let us say the child is seven or eight -- I would superimpose a third party having no interest in the research, no interest in the researcher or his success or failure in his research, in order to obtain that consent in addition to the consent of the parent.

DENNIS SAVER: I am a student at the Medical College of Pennsylvania. Given that risks in human experimentation are unavoidable, even if the risks should be equally distributed among the population, it is axiomatic that the risk will precipitate upon some subjects of experimental procedures. The question then arises of to what degree the researchers and society as a whole bear responsibility towards those unlucky enough to suffer unexpected, untoward effects?

If continuing or even lifelong medical care is needed for treatment of these iatrogenic ills, should the patient pay the cost from his or her own pocket? Obviously the failure to disclose the origin of the illness to the subjects in the case study we have seen this afternoon is indefensible; but it is not even clear in this study whether all subjects who experienced peripheral neuropathy were given continued treatment or if this was free of charge. Is the concept of a national insurance risk pool or some variety of no-fault insurance desirable or a practical remedy in this case? And in the meantime, what is the responsibility of the physician investigator to patients afflicted with unfortunate sequelae to experiments? Although I would have preferred to inflict this question on a more complacent panel, perhaps Mr. Smith would care to respond.

EISENBERG: Before Mr. Smith does, I would agree to absolutely complete and total coverage. And I would like to extend it to the notion that if someone is the unfortunate victim of a medical misfortune -- that is, an anesthetic death not because the anesthetist was incompetent, a depression of blood marrow in the perfectly appropriate use of a drug -- that that individual ought to be compensated whether the doctor did the right thing or not, by a no-fault kind of arrangement. If the doctor did the wrong thing, he ought to be prosecuted in court. And the notion of getting compensation depending upon demonstrating that the doctor was incompetent seems to me to avoid it.

Now I have been very much concerned that there is not, to the best of my knowledge, an adequate policy in research institutions to cover the consequences of untoward effects on the subjects even after everything else has been done right and they knew what they were doing. Why should they be victimized, especially when they volunteered for such a drug?

SMITH: I am not sure that I remember all the questions encompassed in that question -- one of them had to do with compensating victims. I don't know if the insurance industry will ever rise to that occasion. I suspect not, and I am told by people at NIH that they will not. Certainly I think the federal government has an obligation to provide no-fault type insurance where people are injured as the result of research.

I think you alluded to the question of distributing the risks of research. Dr. Eisenberg and I, I think, would part company on that, as well as on a number of other things. I would not agree with his randomized, noninformed consent health insurance scheme. I would prefer to take a first step before that and to exclude from all medical research that is not therapeutic to the individual institutionalized persons and children, unless it is absolutely essential that the research be performed on that particular population and can't be performed on another population.

106

HALPERN: Let me just add two brief observations. First of all, there
is the subject that we have not discussed explicitly: research
sponsored by drug companies for commercial purposes. Typically
these drug tests are designed for submission to the Food and Drug
Administration in support of new drug applications. HEW has ample
jurisdiction to impose the kinds of limitations on that research
process just as if these were research undertakings sponsored by
HEW, and I think it reasonably clear that they should do so. However, in revising their proposed regulations to govern research,
they have excluded research done for submission to the FDA. In the
first draft they had included it, and in the second draft they excluded it.

The point you are making with regard to an insurance requirement
seems to me to be particularly appropriate where you are dealing
with research sponsored by a drug company for commercial purposes.
Such companies should be under a statutory or administrative duty to
assure any iatrogenic damage done by the experiment designed was
insured.

MICHAEL HAMILTON: I am a canon at the Washington Cathedral, and serve
on the medical board of NIH. The consent form, which has been well
criticized for its inadequacies, has a couple of defects I would
like to comment on, because they seem to me to be in general practice
some of the protocols we have to deal with.

First of all, with regard to placebos, is the advantage offered
to the researcher to hide from the prospective patients that placebos
will be used. This enables more people to be recruited. I think
it is unfair and should not be in any protocols, simply because
some people join in the experimentation in the hope of gaining a new
procedural drug, and they ought to be fully aware that they only
have a 50 percent or less chance of receiving one.

Second is the matter of trust. This particular consent form says,
"My physician has explained to me the procedures to be followed,
identifying those that are experimental..." and the possible discomforts, et cetera. This has already been remarked on, but it
occurs in quite a lot of protocols. I think again there is a misunderstanding of the nature of the consent form, which is partly to
help the patient to understand, but also to be a public disclosure
that the procedures involved are competent and ethical and are so
publicly stated.

This leads me to my third point. There is a great deal said
about patients not being able to understand consent forms, and I
think this is overestimated. A lot of it is true. But even if one
of the patients is prevented from fully understanding the consent
form, then the value of the consent form is there. Is not the very
development of a good consent form on the part of the researchers
involved a reflection upon them and one that insures that the quality
of the experiments themselves will be publicly acceptable?

EISENBERG: I would invite my colleagues on either side to comment on the legal consequences that concern me as a physician: that is, how to get an informed consent form that contains all of the information. Well, how far do you go? Do you list the 1 in 10 risks? The 1 in 100 risks? The 1 in 10,000 risks? The 1 in 100,000 risks? By this time you are on the eighth or ninth page of the informed consent form. You decided on the 1 in 100,000 cutoff, and to your misfortune, or to his misfortune, the individual has a risk not listed on the consent form. I have been told by some attorneys that such an explicit form, failing to contain something that was very remote but nonetheless possible, in fact puts the physician at greater risk than the general form.

   I do think it is highly impractical to think that in the ordinary patient-physician transaction, of which this is one special type, it is logical for the physician to convey to the patient all of the things listed in the drug insert packages that appear. I just don't think that is reasonable in medical practice, but I would like some comments on the legalities of it.

ROBBINS: And reasonableness.

SMITH: I am not prepared to comment on the legality of it. I think I can comment on the reasonableness of it. If I were your patient, or your potential subject, I would hope that you would impart to me before I agreed to participate in your experiment everything that you know about that experiment and the procedures to be used, insofar as you are able to explain it to me in layman's terms. And I think that is what ought to be on the consent form.

EISENBERG: Written down?

SMITH: It would have to be both explained and written down for certain kinds of subjects in certain kinds of experiments supervised by a third party.

HALPERN: This is an evolving area of the law at the present time -- and the law differs from state to state, and probably from judge to judge -- that leaves the researcher in an extremely uncomfortable position, making it all the more important, I think, that he be receiving competent legal advice right from the beginning of the time he begins to design his research protocol. The basic rule, I think, in this area is one of reasonableness, and Bill Smith's formulation is one that would commend itself in many courts.

BARBARA ROSENKRANTZ: I am an historian of science at Harvard. I have been listening to the discussion on informed consent with peculiar feelings that in the name of ethical procedure we were evolving a sense of social responsibility. Somehow or other the informed

108

consent procedure is being looked on as a way of relieving the
researcher and the practitioner of the responsibilities involved in
adequate research development. I don't assume that this is in a
deliberate form in any sense, but it does seem to me that informed
consent does not take care of our social responsibilities. As we
look at experimental problems, primarily in terms of either medical
or surgical investment, we seem to be consistently ignoring the
social context in which that research takes place, the social environment in which the patient lives or the subject is drawn from,
and the enormous importance this has for the outcome of the research
itself. Designing research, in fact, should systematically take
these matters into account.

I want to suggest another criterion that seems to me is necessary
and desirable: that the subject population be drawn from the group at
least risk in other respects -- that is, the least social risk, the
least psychological risk -- from the specific question involved.
Similarly, the subject population should be drawn from that section
with the greatest potential benefit from the specific research being
designed. Now maybe we take those things for granted, but it doesn't
seem to me, looking at certain research protocols, that we do.

I just want to ask Mr. Halpern another question -- maybe ask all
three of you, in one sense. There is somehow or other an assumption
presented in this afternoon's discussion that I find difficult to
accept. This is the notion that the subject finds his lawyer a
better advocate for his needs or her needs than some other part of
the population. I am not particularly clear why one professional
group being substituted for another professional group in fact
achieves the kind of advocacy that we have in mind.

SMITH: I know a lot of doctors, and I know a lot of lawyers. I happen
to be a lawyer, and I am not sure but what I wouldn't rather have
doctors supervise me. But the point is to get representatives of
the subjects of some sort involved in a review process and a consent
process. I don't think either Mr. Halpern or I have suggested that
it ought to be exclusively lawyers.

HALPERN: First, I think your point about informed consent is right and
important. To rely on informed consent and no other kinds of professional and scientific checks is a great abdication of the larger
responsibility. You cannot load too much on informed consent.

As to the questions of lawyers, I think the important point is
that there should be some disinterested advocacy and independent
advice available to potential subjects. I suggested that it might
better be a social worker than a lawyer. And I think social workers
properly trained in advocacy skills and also in biomedical research
might be a very worthwhile population to look to.

ROSENKRANTZ: Can you tell me what your definition of *disinterest* is? That is, I think, where my trouble is. I would rather have an interested advocate than a disinterested one.

HALPERN: I mean disinterested in the sense that the advocates have no interest in the research protocol, but have an interest in furthering the best interests of the subject, unalloyed by any other loyalties -- not weighing, in other words, the interest of this particular subject against humanity in the outcomes of this research.

LEWIS THOMAS: I am a little worried about the case report on which much of the discussion has been based. I recall having been told several times that it is hypothetical. As pediatric illnesses carry more last names of pediatricians than is true elsewhere in medicine, and I would therefore not be surprised to be told that there is such a thing as Haym's Syndrome.

EISENBERG: There is not.

THOMAS: Well, there it is. I sort of like to see a hypothetical case report presented, if you can do so, because of there being something very typical about it. I assumed when I read that thing through that somewhere in the country this must have happened over and over again. And I shared with the speakers not only a rising indignation about the events contained in that description, but I even confess to having thought as you took us through the report that perhaps, by God, it might have happened, and there might be a Haym's Syndrome.

Is it in fact in your view typical of the medical research community in this country that a new drug of unknown toxicity, tested inadequately in animals, never before given to human beings, was in fact, as I think you explicitly said, Mr. Smith, tested in this hypothetical case only to establish toxicity levels? Do you think in real life this sort of thing goes on? Do you know of cases where it has gone on? Is there any basis for this whole rather claptrappy story? And would you like to make a comment on the ethics underlying its writing?

SMITH: There is no such thing as Haym's Syndrome. I just want to correct one thing that you said: the case does not state that the only purpose of the experiment was to determine toxicity. It stated that the investigators failed to disclose that that was one of the purposes of the experiment. The experiment had the dual purpose of determining toxicity and determining benefit and weighing those against each other.

To answer your specific question: if you removed from that hypothetical case two features of it -- first, the use of placebos and the existence of a control group; and second, the use of institutionalized children in a juvenile training school -- the case is 100-percent real and factual and is going on today.

110

THOMAS: Could you be more explicit about that?

SMITH: No, sir.

HALPERN: I would just add that I have seen better research protocols, and I have seen worse.

UNIDENTIFIED: Thank you, gentlemen, for throwing some illumination into this controversy. But I think, Mr. Smith, to require the physician not to be the essential experimenter is another hypothetical case, because I know in my experience of no time, other than casual medical experimentation, when the researcher has not become a physician to the subject in the true and total sense of the word. It is only thus that it goes beyond what appears in the consent form or is explained in the protocol or what is done personally in this interrelationship on a true physician-to-patient sense that exists between the subject of the experiment and the scientific investigator.

STUART SPICKER: I am from the University of Connecticut School of Medicine. My field is philosophy, but that doesn't matter today. We have had surgeons speaking on the history of medicine and lawyers speaking on philosophy. That fits Renée Fox's goal, I think, as a beginning.

Now everyone is worried about federal interventions, and I guess we have to turn that moratorium around. That is part of the political motif of this meeting, and that is all right. But it seems to me that we have to get down to the question of machinery. So far, as with the jury system, all we have got are these review committees now federally mandated, even mandated with consent that there will be nonuniversity people on university committees. I sympathize with the problem of special institutions that cannot functionally be built, if you will, like a university committee can be. Having sat on one, I must confess that the mystique I have had about science, never mind about medicine, has all dwindled. It seems to me that the real problems come up so obviously. Since it is experimentation, the researcher has to admit his limits and hence has to translate the complicated concepts in biochemistry into something even he can understand because he is trying to learn more. This is in the best sense. Everyone else on the committee isn't really stupid, and they in fact do understand what a given study is about. They in fact can understand a study of enuresis requiring children to participate. They can understand, when they are given a fairly clear picture from the scientist and the clinician and the other people in the committee, just basically what the chances are of progress in an area.

I can only question one point, therefore, of Dr. Eisenberg's presentation. I think he shows a failing to the power of reason, not only in academe but elsewhere, in the citizenry. I think we have to return to a political motif in Locke and others regarding the trust and reason of human beings, certainly in collection, rather than taking the experimenter protocol per se. Many of the experimenters whom we have dealt with in our own institution simply didn't know that something was important to think about. It is hard to cover every fact. No one is perfect. And each member of these committees has often lent help to others. That maybe is not the finest machinery, but I hope we never return to the privacy of the experimental problematics unless we also turn to only auto-experimentation. That certainly would make sense to me.

I hope that I have helped to focus at least one specific issue: back to the machinery and precisely the debate about the so-called peer groups or peer review committees and their importance rather than their deletion from the system. It is not the federal government anymore when twenty people sit around a table on a problem, respecting the points of view of each other, and have to come to sometimes a very difficult decision.

EISENBERG: I didn't hear myself say that the investigator ought to be autonomous and independent of the peer review committee.

I would further suggest the need to look experimentally and investigatively at systems for controlling and investigating the experimental process. I would like to know, after six months or twelve months or eighteen months of this or that review mechanism, whether in fact it worked, and not only what studies were done and whether they were ethical or not, but what studies were not done. There is a very serious problem in the bureaucratization of anything, and it is the problem the government faces constantly. If you are a bureaucrat and you refuse to let something happen, nobody knows what good might have happened had you permitted it. But if in fact you say yes and a drug is released on the market with perfectly good judgment based on the data available at the time, and then some untoward effect shows up, you are obviously culpable. Consequently, there is a tendency built into the system to avoid being caught off base by taking the conservative position. No one has to look overall at what the costs and deficits on both sides are.

HALPERN: One enormous step forward, it would seem to me, would be for somebody to start to collect, index, and publish decisions of peer review committees so that a kind of common law process could develop by which review committees in Michigan might learn from physicians in New York. Perhaps through that process some norms of acceptable practice might evolve.

ROBBINS: This suggestion has been made before. Has anything actually happened in regard to this? Is it in fact being done? Does anybody here know?

SMITH: I was just going to ask if there was anybody here who is a member of a review group that regularly publishes or allows the public to see the results of its deliberations? Is there any such thing anywhere in the country?

HUGH FUDENBERG: I think this reflects the gap between the biomedical community and those elsewhere in the audience. I am glad the gap has been revealed. Most people in biomedical investigation are in it because they want to do something first. If these deliberations of the review committee -- which in all the institutions I know is composed of laymen, including theologians, et cetera -- were to be published, they would have to publish the purpose and other documentation as well. And this would not necessarily even be a new drug. I would think that the vast majority of people doing something for the first time would refuse to do it if this were the case.

I would also like to point out that on one review committee that I know, the same sort of thing was raised by another attorney. He says that if this drug has never been used before, it would have to be for an exotic form of cancer. Therefore it can't be done. To him research from that point is to see what has been done before with any complications. I think there is a great gap. Most investigators by research do not mean doing something that has been done before.

FRED HIATT: I work with the Children's Defense Fund. I wish to make a comment on Dr. Thomas's doubting that this case could have happened. His faith in the research profession is fairly typical of the faith that a lot of scientists have in their own professions, and I think it is this faith that is in large part responsible for vigilance being less careful than it could be. In fact, as Mr. Smith said, this case pretty much did happen and is happening. This may not be the norm, but certainly I think anybody who is here from a research review committee would say that unsatisfactory consent is not at all unusual, and more serious abuses do certainly happen.

I think that the point is not how commonplace these abuses are. A lot of people today said, well, why are we worrying? These subspecies are just needles in the haystacks. Most research is beneficial and ethical, so what is the problem? That may or may not be true. I tend to think there are more abuses than reach the newspaper or congressional committees. Even if they were just needles in the haystack, when you talk about revising regulation and procedure for the protection of subjects, it is these abuses that you have to keep in mind, not polio vaccines. Is it possible, given a lot of the anxieties we have heard here today, to develop regulations that will prevent the abuses, which certainly are occurring, without impeding pediatric research?

SMITH: I think it is possible, and I think HEW started on that road when they originally published proposed regulations for the protection of children involved in research. Those regulations, for example, contained the proposal for child consent, or at least child approval for nontherapeutic research when a child was over seven.

They contained a prohibition on research on parentless children.
They made a stab at the institutionalized children process research
problem. They also tried to superimpose on the present review system a couple of other mechanisms. One was an ethical review at the
NIH level, and another was a subject protection committee controlled
by nonresearchers at the institutional level. Because there is a
big hassle going on now at HEW headquarters about these child regulations, it remains to be seen what they are going to look like when
they come out, hopefully within a few weeks or months. But my suspicion is that all those reforms are going to go down the drain
because there has been so much opposition to them. They received
some six hundred comments on those regulations on prisoners,
children, and the mentally infirm, and I think there weren't more
than twenty-five that were categorized as advocates on behalf of
protection or further protections of the subjects.

So my answer to the question is yes, I think it is possible, but
I am not sure HEW is going to end up doing it.

ROBBINS: I would agree that it is possible we are moving toward it.
But let us look at the regulations and their toxicity. There is a
law in Massachusetts that forbids research on a fetus scheduled for
abortion but permits therapeutic research on a viable fetus that may
come to term. This means that the only way one finds out whether
a fetoscope is safe to use is by potentially killing or damaging
fetuses, rather than by using it on a fetus that is going to be
aborted and would have given us the information to use it safely,
if safe it can be. Now that is my idea of a kind of regulation
that in the name of morality is obscene. I would just urge that we
not multiply formal rules that do not, in fact, have the likelihood
of controlling the misbehavior we would like to regulate.

BERNARD DAVIS: I am a professor of microbiology at Harvard and a former
professor of pharmacology. I would like to come back to a point
raised by the two members of the legal profession on the panel. As
I understand it, the legal process for a very long time in this
country has been fundamentally a necessary process, with attorneys
for the two contending sides presenting their arguments as forcibly
as possible for each. There are many other important processes in
our society where decisions are traditionally not reached by an adversary process.

The teacher-student relation is theoretically a nonadversary
process, although it seems to be coming more of one these days. The
search for some kind of an objective truth by scientists involves
arguments but not fundamentally an adversary process. And the relation between the physician and his patient has not traditionally been
an adversary process.

I appreciate very much Mr. Halpern's suggestion that what we need
is an effort to achieve more collaboration in institutions that
would promote more collaboration between the medical profession and

114

other interested groups in improving the standards of ethics in
medical experimentation. I am a little worried by the danger that
since this is initiated by people who have become much concerned
over the very real excesses that have occurred, the abuses that have
occurred in more or less instances in medical research, what is
arising may have much too much of the adversary process in it to
yield the kind of really cooperative collaborative arrangement that
we would, I think, all like to see. I am afraid that if it becomes
the medical profession confronted by public interest lawyers supported by wide public appeal, which is very easy to generate and
has already been generated over the kinds of issues we are discussing, we may end up with great damage to the quality of medical research and the quality of medical care in this country.

To illustrate what I mean by the adversary process, let me ask
Mr. Smith if there wasn't more than a hint of advocacy in the very
case that he presented? First he described the experiment as nontherapeutic. I would like to have him define what he meant by
therapeutic, since these subjects were given a drug that on the
basis of animal experimentation offered very real promise of arresting the progress of the disease. More important is the way he
described the role of the physicians in violating the Hippocratic
Oath by engaging in an experiment clearly designed to advance the
interest of the investigators and not that of the subjects. Now if
these subjects were suffering from a disease that reached the mortality of 40 percent by the age of forty, and if animal experiments
gave real promise of arresting the progress of the disease, and if
no other promising therapy was available, I would like an explanation of why this is violating the Oath of Hippocrates; or more important, if it is not, why did he so interpret it?

SMITH: First of all, I confess to being an advocate, I confess to
advocating here, and I am proud of it. I hope that the speakers who
went before me would admit that they too are advocates, including
the three this morning, and those on the panel on the fetus.

Let me address the question of therapeutic research. I had the
privilege of participating in a group that wrestled with some of
the problems that HEW tried to resolve in writing the outlines for
protecting children in medical experimentation, and the toughest
problem was trying to define what was beneficial and what was not
beneficial research. When you try to make rules or regulations or
even make statements in this area, you always seem to get back to
what is therapeutic and what isn't therapeutic. Therapeutic seems
to be a reasonable test of some things that should or shouldn't be
done or the procedures that are going to be imposed.

I would say that therapeutic research is research that is undertaken for the primary purpose of treating a physical or mental illness in an individual patient and that if successful would reasonably
be expected to alleviate substantially the individual's condition.
I would enclose a test as part of that definition. I would say that

if there were no other possible benefit from the procedure, the physician would immediately undertake the procedure for the patient's benefit. So with the imposition of that definition and that test as therapeutic research, I would say all this research is not therapeutic. When I suggested a child's consent and suggested that doctors shouldn't experiment on their own patients, I tied those suggestions to nontherapeutic research and was using in my own mind that definition.

ROBBINS: Would this include vaccine trials where, assuming that the vaccine were effective, the patient would be benefited?

SMITH: This is where it is very difficult to write the rules and definitions.

ROBBINS: You gave me my answer.

UNIDENTIFIED: There were forty subjects in this trial. Twenty of them got placebos; therefore only twenty got the drug. Fifty percent of those receiving the drug suffered a severe adverse reaction. Only the six who continued to exhibit that condition were given follow-up care. Why was the other remaining population not given continuing care or at least periodic examinations to see if they were going to come up with that adverse reaction at a later time?

ROBBINS: I think that can be quite simply answered.

MICHAEL WAITZKIN: I am at the Yale Law School. I would like to return to a comment that was made several turns back that seemed to slip by unnoticed and that I thought was relatively important. This was in regard to the discussion of whether the decisions of the peer review committee should be published to develop some sort of common law and to develop some generally acceptable provisions on ethical standards. The gentleman who responded to that question said something that was rather important. It seemed to me that what he was saying was that the intense competition between scientists in his view would preclude the publication of such reports. This level of intense competition among scientists, as reflected in that comment, is not always compatible with the interests of the recipients of the care that they are giving, the subject in the experiment, or compatible at all necessarily with the development of general ethical principles. This is the point raised, and I think it reflects something that other people have said: the groups that have been on the stage today tend to be compatible among themselves and incompatible perhaps with the interest of the audience. If we had had that gentleman on the stage with these gentlemen, I think that point could have been raised more easily and the concept been more clearly articulated.

116

UNIDENTIFIED: There seems to be a great concern about the possibility of the kind of collaboration that has been so often suggested here. I wish to submit that perhaps we are thinking of ourselves as much too special. I don't think the subject of ethics and morality of human experimentation, on which I have worked so many years, is really so different from some of the problems that communities have tackled in education, housing, social welfare, environment and the like. I think, frankly, that many of us -- and I exclude myself at this point -- distrust the public; and the reasons that we aren't making the committees fully knowledgeable about these things, or even having committees in some cases, is that we don't really want them to have this information. We talk about it, but we haven't really set up methods to make this possible or available. If the same kind of interest and campaigning and the same kind of selling, if you will, that has been done in the fields I have mentioned were done in this one, I think the problem would be substantially lessened and reduced. We would have the kind of general and, I hope, useful and constructive criticism that we claim we want.

If we really do, then let us see whether there are not methods well known to all of us that can be applied here. That would, of course, include that we have joint activity among the professions and the others, teaching and training; that we perhaps make available all kinds of seminars and the like, not just of this kind but throughout the country, and open the various committees that presumably are setting up the standards that we have. This would also, I think, take some of the bite off the need for regulation if we are willing to accept community determinations. They are not all going to be good. Some of them are going to be very bad, but I think it is worth trying, and if necessary we will live with some of those and turn to education, turn to publicity, if you will, turn to all the techniques we are familiar with to try to get the kind of right decisions we claim we want.

ROBBINS: Thank you. Does the panel wish to make any final comment?

EISENBERG: Well, I would wholeheartedly concur that in the end it is society or those people who have the power in society who will determine what science is and what science does, and what physicians are able to do.

One of the elements of unreality in this discussion is the failure to identify some of the forces in some of the reasons for the attacks on science, part of which thinks that scientists have done what they shouldn't and have characteristics that they pretend they don't have. But it is also true that there are a variety of reasons for turning in a mindless way when those forces that have been identified as a source of evil in society make them a much easier target than looking at the political forces that distorted the potential progress of society. When one looks at the kind of lovely issues that get discussed at an ethical level, particularly in fetal research, one also understands that some of the opposition to fetal research has little to do with the ethics of anything other than the ethics of abortion as it is perceived in some people's minds. That is why Edelin is getting it. The connection between Edelin and the so-called grave-robbing case is that they all came out of the same contacts. Who is being denied the care? The black and the poor, and I think that ought to be put into the context of this discussion, too.

HALPERN: The notion of the attacks on science as being a framing concept in which you should deal with these ethical issues we have been airing is, I think, a very grave mistake and one that I have seen repeated all too often. I had the experience with one very good research scientist who came to defend an indefensible research protocol -- considerably worse, Dr. Thomas, than what we have set out here -- simply, he told me, because he felt that science was under attack everywhere and that it should be defended on the beaches and in the mountains.

If we are going to have the kind of collaboration some of us have discussed, it is going to be only on the basis of shared concerns and shared values, not on a conceptualization that looks to science and its attackers and defenders.

ROBBINS: I want to thank you all for being here. There have been some obvious deficiencies in our system, but, as our Forum pointed up, nothing is ever perfect. On the other hand, there has been some considerable discussion of important issues, discussion that I hope we will continue in the spirit that has existed here.

DAY II

DAY II
AN OVERVIEW

Lewis Thomas
Chairman

It was, in my view, a useful Forum, and I am glad it was held, but I
hope fervently that there will not be another one. The chief value of
this exercise was in its demonstration that you cannot settle a problem
of such complexity by calling in representatives of two, already quite
polarized, points of view and instructing them to discuss the problem
as though it were a matter of principle.

I suppose it is, after all, a matter of principle -- in the sense
that you can always line up two opposing sides, one asserting that human
research is always, under whatever circumstances, an unqualified social
evil, the other affirming, just as flatly, that it is quite generally a
good endeavor. Indeed, we came near to this degree of polarization at
several points in the Forum, and the discussion led nowhere beyond the
confrontation.

I emerged from the sessions with a different viewpoint. Principle
or no, the questions before the Forum turned out to be matters of
extraordinary *detail*, and there is really no way to conduct a broad discussion in two days when the details are all so crucially important,
and especially when none of the participants had anything like hard,
analytical information concerning the detail.

Most of the bits of detailed information that I now feel the need
for are actually lacking on my side of the fence. As an old defender
of the importance and value of clinical research, it embarrasses me that
I know so little, factually, about how satisfactorily and safely the
present system works. I do not really know for sure that the review
committees in all hospitals, or even in some, provide total protection
against trivial research, research for the sake of writing papers, research carrying some hazard for the subjects, or research holding no
promise of benefit for anyone. I *think* the system works well, as seen

121

firsthand in the teaching hospitals I've known, but I really cannot prove anything beyond the hunch and the obvious wish. This was rather effectively pointed out on several occasions by the Forum participants opposed to today's system.

Therefore, I conclude that there is a rather urgent need for someone to make a new study. I am aware of the books already written, and the evidence presented, much of it anecdotal and placing great emphasis on individual instances of conspicuous sin, notably the Alabama syphilis study. I still feel the need for much more information. I suggest that the matter be placed before the Institute of Medicine, with the suggestion that this organization authorize a full-scale panel of experts, representing all sides of the issue, to conduct a study, at first hand, of the review mechanisms, protective rules, approved criteria, et cetera, in a meaningful sample of the teaching hospitals of this country.

By information in detail I mean such matters as the size and composition of the review committees, number and length of meetings held in the past year, number of projects reviewed, number approved and rejected. It would be of special interest to have detailed information about the rejected category, since this might provide clues as to the existence of real hazards in today's system.

I was alarmed by some of the charges of injustice, inhumanity, and coldness made at various points in the Forum, and it seemed to me that American medicine would be in deep trouble for its future if these were shown to be generally true. I cannot believe that the teaching hospitals are up to the sorts of mischief alluded to, nor so lacking in effective mechanisms for the surveillance of their own clinical research. But I would like to know what the facts of the matter really are.

WELCOME

Donald S. Fredrickson
President
Institute of Medicine

I am privileged to serve on the General Advisory Committee of the Academy Forum. At a recent Committee meeting another medical member, Dr. Frederick Robbins, and I were guilty of setting up a rhetorical fuss with the other members of the Committee, who represent the variety of disciplines within the National Academy of Sciences. *Why*, we asked, when portions of the world are faced with imminent starvation, when we are down to the last half-century or perhaps quarter-century of the use of fossil fuels for all time, when we seem to be spraying away the only ozone layer that we are ever likely to have, when in most of our great urban centers the systems for mass transit and for the administration of criminal justice seem to be vying with each other for honors in inadequacy -- why, in the face of all this, does the Committee spend so much time discussing more provocative medical topics for future forums?

This, I confess, was a sham. The obvious answer was written in the faces and in the words of yesterday's session, ever groping for the meaning of life. We have found a subject of great and continuing fascination and certain extraordinary importance in the question of what man is doing to man in the interest of humanity and through the medium of science. Some of these most intensely personal interactions fall under the rubric of medicine and biomedical research. If they sometimes involve abstractions, they are universal ones: the beginning of human life; the end of it; and in between, a great unknown that differs from some of the other voids out there on the rim of human perceptions. For this biomedical void is constantly being filled by human endeavor, and with each turn of new knowledge and new technique comes another problem and another tough decision to be made.

It is small wonder that such decisions are not left for a single profession to make on behalf of us all, and it is no wonder that they cry

123

124

for open and constant debate. The conflict of values inherent in medicine and in the whole health care dilemma have special interest for that body of the Academy known as the Institute of Medicine. At least half of the participants in yesterday's Forum sessions included Institute members or others who have been involved in its activities. The provisions of the charter and the pattern of enrollment of participants in its activities reflect the great diversity of professions, of institutions, and of opinions that are involved in dealing with health as a public issue. The Institute of Medicine is in one sense a continuing forum, regularly engaged in the kind of ecumenical debate and the balancing of tensions that are characteristic of this two-day meeting.

Recently the Institute has received a generous grant from the Andrew W. Mellon Foundation to structure and examine some of the critical ethical choices that are posed by a wide range of public policy decisions concerning health practices; and it is of note that among the activities proposed are several that were discussed here yesterday, including the compilation of a record of the decision-making process that might help guide further decisions in informed consent and experimental procedures.

Many of you will take back to your own institutions a desire to implement ways to answer some of the questions that will be unanswered after this Forum. And so too, the Institute of Medicine will attempt to knit further the raveled sleeve of these discussions, which now begin again.

INDIVIDUAL NEEDS vs. SOCIETAL BENEFITS

How Are the Risks Distributed?

THE MILITARY / THE PRISONER

Albert B. Sabin
Alvin J. Bronstein
William N. Hubbard, Jr.

ALBERT SABIN

I will make my points briefly at the beginning and then document them
to the extent that time permits.
1. Some of the most important preventive and therapeutic products
in current use in human medicine could not have been developed without
the use of adult human volunteers in nontherapeutic medical research,
that is, research on persons who do not have the disease or disorder
under study and are not in immediate danger of acquiring it.
2. The ongoing need for such volunteers from armed forces, prison,
and other population groups is as great as ever for acquiring the knowledge needed for the eventual control and optimum treatment of important
infectious and other diseases.
3. Personal experience and the dispassionate observations of
others -- by this I mean those who are not themselves engaged in biomedical research on volunteers -- testify to the important personal
gratifications that the majority of adult volunteers derive from the
justifiable conviction that their participation contributes knowledge
that cannot be otherwise obtained for the elimination or relief of human
suffering or in the case of the armed forces volunteers from providing
the knowledge needed for the optimum management of the hygienic, nutritional, stress, health, and other problems -- and here I want to indicate especially problems that are peculiar to service in the armed
forces.
4. Consent without coercion is implicit in the word *volunteer*.
Coercion in the sense of enforcing or bringing about consent by force or
threat, as is well described in the Nuremberg Code, is not part of the
American system of recruitment of human beings for service as subjects

in medical research, and contemporary critics of this system do not have this type of coercion in mind. The issue centers around a more subtle type of coercion, more along the lines of seduction, involving opportunities for temporary escape from boredom and unpleasant surroundings (for example, those in prison) or undesirable activities (for example, some military duties) and offers of modest financial gain not otherwise available to the volunteer.

The conclusion that no man is a free agent in prisons or in the armed forces and that accordingly the expression consent without coercion is impossible under these conditions is based, in my judgment, on an untenable definition of coercion involving the same subtle factors that influence so-called freedom of choice in almost everyone's life. For instance, I may want to punch somebody in the nose. Maybe before this symposium is over I will feel like it. But the law restrains me. I do not have that much free choice. I want to do many other things. I want to cross the street against the red light. I am in a hurry. The law says if I do it and I am caught, I will have to pay the price. So we are all constrained by certain limitations on our free choice and I maintain that the free choice involved in volunteering falls within the same category. It is not identical among those serving in the armed forces and in prison.

5. There are some very good people, who, because of their sincere concern for the protection of human freedom, oppose medical experiments on human volunteers in prisons as part of their justifiable wish to reform the penal system. But I think they are misguided because:

(a) it is the least objectionable aspect of the current penal system, if it is objectionable at all, and its elimination would have very little impact on bringing about the more truly desirable and urgent changes, and

(b) it would eliminate something that, in the judgment of others who are also concerned with the protection of human freedom including prisoners, [1]is highly beneficial for the vast majority of those who volunteer.

6. You have all heard about the Nuremberg Code and Declaration of Helsinki. I would like to introduce a Sabin Bill of Rights in this particular issue. I would like to propose that the right to volunteer for medical experiments, carried out under properly supervised and enforced guidelines and conditions, is one of the human rights that should not be denied to anyone because of service in the armed forces, imprisonment for a crime against society, unemployment, poverty, boredom, or even a sincere desire to help others. That is a right that should not be denied to anyone.

During the first session of this Forum, Dr. Lewis Thomas discussed the benefits of research with humans. I should like to emphasize here several benefits and briefly describe some personal experiences with army, prisoner, and medical student volunteers.

Dr. Franklin A. Neva of the National Institutes of Health recently pointed out that:

> The fact that physicians, not only in the United States, but all over the world, can treat malaria in as rational a pharmacologic fashion as they do is largely the result of malaria volunteer research programs that have existed for the last 30 years...The malaria program of the National Institutes of Health at the Atlanta Federal Penitentiary has recognized and, we believe, has fulfilled the highest standards of medical ethics in clinical research by obtaining truly informed consent, by exerting no direct or indirect coercion, by having a record of minimal risks (e.g., no deaths in more than 4,000 infections since the 1940s), and by producing results of great medical importance.[2]

Extensive malaria volunteer research programs have also been carried out under the auspices and with the financial support of the U.S. Army Medical Research and Development Command since World War II. The continuing emergence of drug-resistant varieties of malarial parasites and the need to explore possibilities of active immunization against malaria will require ongoing experiments with human volunteers under conditions of strict isolation and ongoing observations such as are uniquely available in prisons.

The recent extraordinary advances in our understanding of viral hepatitis would have been impossible without the infrastructure of knowledge and the banks of specimens -- serum specimens, stool specimens -- acquired from studies on human subjects during the decades since World War II. Moreover, if suitable candidate vaccines should emerge from current exploratory studies on chimpanzees and monkeys, the ultimate decision regarding their suitability and effectiveness in human beings will be possible only after careful, stepwise studies on human subjects under strict conditions of isolation.

The ultimate control of epidemics and pandemics of influenza rests on past, present, and future studies on human subjects under carefully controlled and isolated conditions.

My own experience dates back to World War II and includes medical students who volunteered for studies on a vaccine against Japanese encephalitis and others later, that is, after the war, on a vaccine against Dengue Fever. It includes studies on prisoners at the New Jersey State Prison at Trenton who served as subjects for basic studies on Dengue and Sandfly Fevers, and about twenty-two years ago on hundreds of prisoners at the Federal Reformatory at Chillicothe, Ohio, who served as subjects for basic studies on various attenuated polio virus strains that ultimately led to the selection of the strains currently used throughout the world for the preparation of the live attenuated polio virus vaccine administered by mouth.

My first assignment on arrival in Egypt in early 1943 was to determine the relative effectiveness of British and U.S. repellents against the sandflies that transmit Phlebotomus Fever. This disease was reported to have rendered noneffective about 70 percent of the British

130

forces during Rommel's first successful attack on Tobruk, and was known
to be prevalent in Italy, which was still under Nazi occupation. American military personnel, including myself, and one British colonel
served as volunteers in these tests that were carried out along the Dead
Sea in Palestine, the only place where we could catch thousands of sandflies at that time of the year.

The available time does not permit me to analyze the variety of motivations I encountered in individual volunteers, but there is no doubt
in my mind that the desire to be of service to others was a dominant motive and that the majority of volunteers derived their greatest gratifi-
cation from the feeling that they had done something good for others.

My own impressions are fortified by those of others not personally
involved in the direction of such experiments. To cite only a few: the
1974 article, "Prisoners as Laboratory Subjects," by Dr. Norvell Morris
and Mr. Michael Mills of the Center for Studies in Criminal Justice of
the University of Chicago Law School[1]; the very recent report of the
Fordham-Yale Prison Research Group entitled, "Pharmacological Testing in
a Correctional Institution"[3]; and an article entitled, "$20-a-Day Guinea
Pigs with a Nose for Medical Research" by H. Lawrence Lack.[4]

I am not saying that some research on prisoners in some prisons is
bad and should be corrected. I frankly do not know. All I can say is
that the situations under which I worked showed how well it could be
done. Moreover, there was no breaking of the Nuremberg Code, there was
no coercion, and it was very beneficial to the prisoners themselves. If
I were interested in the welfare of prisoners, I would give those of
them who desire to participate the privilege, the right, to do it and
not prevent them from having that opportunity.

ALVIN BRONSTEIN

I believe that the presentations so far have been rather vague, with no
clear positions taken. No one has attempted to describe or define informed consent. No one has mentioned the use of captive populations in
human experimentation; and no one has mentioned the state's involvement
except with respect to the regulations concerning medical experimentation, but not with respect to the control of the subject population.
Finally, no one has mentioned the Constitution.

I would therefore like to start my presentation by stating some very
definite positions with respect to the use of prisoners for nontherapeutic medical experimentation.

1. I do not challenge generally the ethics of the experimeter. I do
not believe that is terribly relevant to the major issues except, of
course, for the occasional abuse. If we cannot agree that there have
been published reports[1] of occasional abuses in medical research and drug
testing -- for example, untreated syphilis victims, incidents of hepatitis in state prison systems, and injection of live cancer cells into
patients without their knowledge or consent and without the knowledge

131

and consent of their doctors -- then there would be no point in further dialogue.

It is not so much the actual, occasional abuse of captive human subjects, but the potential for abuse which concerns me. And it is the potential for abuse combined with the state's control in prisons that is of most concern.

2. I do not challenge the fact that some of the most important products in current use in human medicine have been developed with the use of human adults who allegedly volunteered.

3. I do not challenge the need for human subjects on a continuing basis in the future.

4. I do not challenge the fact that there is some amount of coercion that influences every decision that men and women make throughout their lives.

5. I do not claim that prisoners have no right to volunteer.

6. I do not challenge the use of prisoners in medical experiments as part of, to quote Dr. Sabin, a "justifiable wish to reform the penal system." I am not interested in reforming the penal system. The penal system in this country is a cancer on our society. I know of no doctors who are trying to reform cancer; they are trying to eliminate it.

7. My position with respect to the use of prisoners in nontherapeutic medical experimentation is simple and clear; the *de facto* environment of prisons is such that you cannot create an institution in which informed consent without coercion is feasible.[2] Given the nature of the institution of prisons, and the degree of intrusion on the individual, his body and his mind, which necessarily results from nontherapeutic medical experimentation, the constitutional rights of the individual prisoner to be free from invasions of privacy, free from invasions of his human dignity, free from cruel and unusual punishment, and free from injurious state action without due process are violated.

The most important thing that distinguishes the use of captive populations as human subjects from all others is the involvement of the state. The state has possession of, and delivers to the scientist, bodies over which it has control. In an earlier debate Dr. Sabin expressed outrage at my saying that the state delivers bodies to the scientist and particularly objected to the use of the word *bodies*. I am sorry that the use of this word upsets him, but I believe that it is a fair and accurate characterization. The state has total control over the prisoner and creates the conditions of coercion that I will discuss shortly. Furthermore, every commitment order I have ever seen contains the language that the "body of the defendant shall be delivered" to whoever the particular custodian is. I would like to illustrate the degree of state control over a prisoner by quoting to you the official position taken by the United States in a brief filed by the Solicitor General in the Supreme Court of the United States this past January. This case did not deal with medical experimentation, but rather with the claimed arbitrary transfer of prisoners from one institution to another. In illustrating that the prisoner had no right to protest his transfer, the government said:

132

...[t]he very fact of his conviction for a crime, and the legitimate placement of his person into the hands of a custodian who will be responsible for his safekeeping and the supervision of the most intimate details of his life, removes from the prisoner any legitimate expectation that he will be able to control the conditions of his confinement.[5]

I would now like to discuss informed consent as a legal doctrine. We must keep in mind that it is necessarily a flexible doctrine. Obviously there will be differences between informed consent for a mental patient or a prisoner and for a college student in the free world who volunteers for an experiment. But it must always consist of three elements: competency, knowledge, and voluntariness.

The Nuremberg Code, in defining voluntary consent, which the Code indicates is absolutely essential before you may experiment on a human subject, states in pertinent part:

...that the person involved...should be so situated as to be able to exercise free power of choice without the intervention of any element of force, fraud, deceit, duress, over-reaching, or other ulterior form of constraint or coercion and should have sufficient knowledge and comprehension of the elements of the subject matter involved as to enable him to make an understanding and enlightened decision....

I would like to give you an example of the state's involvement in experimentation with prisoners and the state's version of informed consent. The Patuxent Institution in Maryland is a maximum security institution for prisoners who are civilly committed there as "defective delinquents" for an indeterminate sentence up to life. In response to recent claims that prisoners, who are euphemistically referred to as patients at Patuxent, were being forced to participate in drug studies, the governing boards at Patuxent just two weeks ago issued the following report:

Forced Participation in Drug Studies. The Joint Boards find no evidence that participation by patients in drug studies within the Institution was forced. All drug studies conducted within the Institution must first be approved by the Governing Board...All patients were told that participation was on a voluntary basis; and those who did participate gave their informed consent to the extent that informed consent is possible in an institutional setting. No doubt many patients were motivated to participate in the drug study by the money they received for their participation and by the expectation that their participation would benefit them within the Institution. The Joint Boards do not believe that the presence of these factors makes a patient's participation in a drug study forced. Furthermore, there is no evidence that a patient's participation in a drug study actually does improve his chances for early release or in any way

affects his progress within the Institution. Nevertheless, it is
difficult to see how these factors which affect a patient's choice
to participate in a drug study can be entirely eliminated because
patients have few opportunities to earn money within the Institution
and generally cannot be disuaded from believing that everything they
do affects their progress in the Institution.[4]

Thus, you see the state, which has control of the prisoners, which
approves the drug studies, which creates the coercion, admitting the
existence of the coercion but denying that there is forced participation
in drug studies.

Let me illustrate the impossibility of a constitutionally valid informed consent -- one made with competence, full knowledge, and voluntariness -- by talking about the quality of prison life. Keep in mind
throughout my description, the important need that was expressed by almost all of the speakers yesterday for openness, exposure, and prohibi-
tions against secrecy when using human subjects. For example, Dr. Moore
said, "Don't work in secret"; and Dr. McDermott said that "The climate
of openness is most important."

Prisons in this country are closed, secret, and inherently coercive
institutions. Control and security are the paramount concerns of the
prison administrators. Rehabilitation of prisoners is neither the goal
nor the practice. More than 90 percent of all the monies budgeted for
corrections in this country goes for control and security. Less than
10 percent of the entire corrections budget in the country goes for the
ridiculous and ineffective programs that exist in some prisons.[5] Most
experiments using prisoners are conducted in medium or maximum security
institutions.[6] These are the institutions where the control is the
closest and most coercive and where conditions are most oppressive.
These are the institutions where the prisoner has the fewest available
options. For example, let us look at the available options to a state
prisoner in Illinois at the maximum security prison at Stateville, where
they are conducting malaria research on prisoners. According to the
last available data from the Law Enforcement Assistance Administration,
a division of the Justice Department, a prisoner in Illinois can earn a
daily wage rate at a regular prison job of from thirty-two to fifty-five
cents. However there are only jobs available for approximately one-
third of the prisoners. On the other hand an Illinois prisoner can
earn fifty dollars a month as a research subject in the malaria tests.[7]
Prison wages generally, or the absence of them, act as a coercive force
in prison life. According to the same LEAA data, six states pay no
prison wages at all, seventeen states pay less than fifty cents a day,
twenty-one states pay between fifty cents and one dollar a day, and six
states pay more than one dollar a day. In those states that do pay
something the estimated percentage of prisoners who earn wages ranges
from 10 percent to 95 percent so that not all prisoners can earn wages
even in those states which pay wages.[8]

The extensive use of indeterminate sentences in this country is
another extremely coercive element in prison life. The prisoner knows

that the date of his release from prison, the single most important
thing in his life, is subject to the whim and caprice of the prison administration as well as his behavior in prison. Pleasing the prison
administration becomes an important element of prison life. And prisoners know the economic advantages to prisons of having drug programs.
The existence of parole boards throughout this country, which make the
single most important decision in a prisoner's life, is another pressure. Even for those prisoners who do not have indeterminate sentences,
his or her release date is still indeterminate in the sense that it is
decided by the parole board.[9]

The barrenness of most of prison life is another factor. Having drug
programs in maximum security institutions helps to continue the existence of these institutions by providing a prisoner one of the few es-
capes from the reality of prison life. If a prisoner were in a community facility or in a very minimum custody facility with a wide range of
available activities he would not use the sometimes painful and sometimes dangerous participation in a drug program as the only escape from
prison life. In a medium or maximum security institution, of the kind
where most medical experimentation on prisoners takes place, the state
exercises total control over every moment of the prisoner's life. The
state tells the prisoner how he must live, when to sleep, when to get
up, when to eat, what to eat, what to do and when to do it, all adding
up to the most oppressive and coercive institution that we have in our
society.

It is my firm belief that having regulations and procedures and review committees will not change this inherent quality of coerciveness,
nor will it make possible a legal informed consent to participate in
medical experimentation. On this point I would again like to quote
from the Solicitor General's brief filed on behalf of the United States
government in the case I mentioned earlier. In discussing why procedural due process before a prisoner is transferred is unnecessary the
government states:

> To a considerable extent, subjection to potentially uninformed
> decision-making is a necessary result of committing an individual to
> a custodian who will control the most minute details of his daily
> life. Realistically, the potential for unfairness, even under the
> most comprehensive procedures, can be eliminated only by eliminating
> the custodial control.[10]

A growing number of people who, next to prisoners, know the quality
of prison life best -- corrections officials -- have come to the same
conclusion about the use of prisoners for medical experiments. A fair
number of states, most recently Pennsylvania, Massachusetts, and
Illinois, have banned the use of prisoners as human subjects because
they recognize the difficulty of obtaining a legal informed consent in
prison. As one corrections official in Oregon put it: "We are not
running a Greek democracy here -- no man is a free agent in prison."[11]

Finally, we have this issue of weighing individual risks against the benefits to society. I think that issue is irrelevant and cannot be ethically reached with you are dealing with prisoners. Again, it is the involvement of the state that makes the potential for abuse so overwhelming that it precludes that issue from consideration. If you agree, as many of you have, that you cannot obtain a totally legal informed consent, then you are permitting the state to be involved in this risk-benefit measuring. Why should we even bother with consent if the benefits to society are great enough? We can pass over the risks to individuals where the state decides it is for the greater good of society. I think that the risk-benefit argument is a very scary and dangerous one when you are dealing with the state's captives.

Let me give you some examples of the power of the state. A few years ago the state of California believed that it had the power to perform lobotomies on "dangerous" prisoners. Indeed, the state of California through its agents, neurosurgeons, exercised that power on a number of prisoners until a public disclosure and adverse publicity brought these experiments to a halt.[12] The state of California believes that it has the power to administer the drug anectine to prisoners with "behavior problems."[13] Anectine is described by prisoners and others as simulating death. Just two years ago the state of Iowa believed that it had the power to administer the drug apomorphine to state prisoners for such violations as refusing to say "Yes, Sir" to prison guards. Apomorphine induces serious nausea and vomiting episodes, and the state of Iowa believed it had that power until the United States Court of Appeals for the Eighth Circuit recently said otherwise.[14] About two years ago the Federal Bureau of Prisons believed that it had the power to transfer thirty-one federal prisoners who were considered serious problem prisoners to an aversive behavior modification program called START at the Federal Medical Center in Springfield, Missouri. A federal court recently ruled that the Bureau acted in violation of the Constitution in making these transfers.[15]

These, of course, are gross examples, but they do illustrate the potential for abuse when the state believes it has the power to measure individual risks against societal benefits. I don't believe the state should have that power in a free and democratic society. I think it is dangerous for prisoners. I think it is dangerous for me and for you.

WILLIAM HUBBARD

We have heard both yesterday and today the reiteration of a dilemma. From the point of view of logic this is important analytically, but it does not arrive in and of itself at any kind of operative solution. The dilemma itself has been well described. However, I would suggest that the problem before us is not to further illuminate by reiteration the dilemma itself, but rather to work toward the solution of the problem of preserving the personal and social benefits of research carried out in settings that are designed to be limiting on freedoms while avoiding the exploitation of the situation of the institutionalized person.

The paradigm of this problem is the prisoner or the common soldier; but students, laboratory workers, and patients in other than private care settings are perfectly valid examples of other groups involved in this same dilemma. It is also worth mentioning that the Nuremberg statement refers to ulterior coercion. In recognizing the moral implications of the logical positivist position, exemplified by such writers as Skinner and Munod, there is a nullification of the legal idea of a free-will decision because every person is ultimately coerced to reach a position because of his genetic heritage and his life experience.

In proposing, then, a means of solution to the problem or a synthesis of the dilemma in Hegelian terms, I will use the example of drug testing in a prison population, directly implying a generalization of the example and proposing a general synthesis of the dilemma.

Dr. Sabin and many others have described the unusual and perhaps unique value of utilizing a prison group living in a defined environment that is subject to control and in which the individual is not penalized by removing him from his alternate activities in order to devote time to an experiment. Since these very same people typically have quite limited opportunity to contribute to the general welfare, participation in efforts carrying large potential social benefits does, in fact, add to their own sense of self-esteem. The opportunity to make the choice of participation, whether by the Sabin statement or less explicit ones, is really an unusual chance for self-determination in a setting where most activity is directed by regulation and authority. These advantages are documented in recent publications.[1,2]

As I understand it, the potential advantages that are available from this kind of investigation are generally accepted, and the dilemma is created by a judgment. This judgment is that whatever the advantages may be, they are counterbalanced by the exploitation of the person of the prisoner. The problem of exploitation has been very well defined by Mr. Bronstein. This definition asserts that the very circumstances of being a prisoner are so highly coercive that a free-will decision is unavailable, that participation is therefore unconstitutional and, among other things, is a form of cruel and unusual punishment. Furthermore, it contends that research protocols may be and have been actually conducted in an inhumane and disrespectful way insofar as human rights are concerned.

The philosophical, ethical, and theoretical aspects of this problem have been widely discussed in both lay and professional publications. I will therefore confine my remarks entirely to an empirical approach to the solution of the problem. This approach is based on almost fifteen years of continuing personal association with the planning, development, and operation of a program of pharmacological testing in humans conducted at Michigan correctional institutions. This actual experience in problem solving constitutes a case study approach to the broader issues involved.

The State Prison of Southern Michigan is the largest walled penal institution in the United States and, indeed, in the world. It is designed for maximum security. It houses approximately 4,400 men, 45 percent

of them white and 55 percent nonwhite. A pool of approximately 745
volunteers now exists, consisting of 67 percent white and 33 percent
nonwhite. The corrections officials in Michigan are progressive, and
provisions for recreational and rehabilitative programs are, in fact,
abundant. Outgoing mail is not opened, and incoming mail is inspected
only for contraband. Inmates have access to telephones any time they
are outside of their cells, which is most of the day. It is not a
pleasant place; but to the extent compatible with the necessary regi-
mentation of life in prisons, the dignity and personal rights of the inmates are preserved. It is this environment, this quality, developed
through the Department of Corrections, that provides the initial feasibility for the proper conduct of clinical research within that correctional institution.

The information regarding the testing programs is distributed at the
time the new inmate is admitted to the institution. This is the only
announcement or recruitment notice that he will receive. He himself
must initiate the writing of a letter to the clinic sponsor in order to
be considered for inclusion as a member of the clinic research panel.

A scale of payments is set by the Department of Corrections and is
adjusted for inconvenience and sometimes discomfort, such as finger
sticks and vena punctures. The sponsors of these programs of research
carry the full liability for any injuries that may occur and for the
medical care and costs for any time the inmate may lose, because of the
experience, in his normal prison occupation. If someone were to engage
in a study that lasted seven days, and this would be somewhat unusual,
the average income for that seven-day period would be about $78.

The proposed protocols are reviewed by a protection committee that
is composed of: two biomedical scientists; three practicing physicians;
two attorneys, one of whom must be and is identified with prisoner advocacy; and one lay member. That committee meets at least every month to
review the activities of the program. Each member of the committee has
veto authority on all decisions; each decision must be unanimous; and a
negative decision cannot be overruled. The Director of the Department
of Corrections himself may overrule any protocol the committee approves.
Any study that is begun may be stopped at any time by the Warden, by
the Director, by the physician responsible for the study, or by the
Clinic Director. Any prisoner may drop out of any study at any time.

In addition to this, there is an administrative review group, which
oversees the policies and activities of the protection committee. This
review group must give unanimous approval to any change in policy.

During the year 1974, twenty-seven protocols were submitted by Upjohn
scientists, and all were finally approved. However, only five of that
twenty-seven were approved as they were submitted. Of those that were
changed, fourteen had to do with changes in the adequacy of informed
consent. This would suggest to me that the reviewers are taking their
responsibility seriously.

Once a protocol has been approved, five or six candidates are likely
to be reviewed in order to select one for participation. The rate of
rejection of the study by the candidates that are offered runs between

10 and 15 percent -- the same as the rate of rejection at the Bronson Hospital Clinical Research Unit in Kalamazoo, where candidates are volunteers from the community for protocols essentially identical with those conducted in the prison.

Since this clinic opened in 1964, 12,000 inmates have participated in drug testing programs. One death occurred in a man who had a stroke. However, when the code was broken it was found that he was a placebo control in a double-blind protocol. I must admit there was a moment of anxiety before the code was broken.

There have been, in addition, nine episodes of illness: five of them were due to spontaneous diseases, three were probably related to the studies, and one remains obscure. All nine of these patients have recovered without sequelae. This record, I would suggest, implies the effectiveness of the efforts of all those concerned with the program. I would agree with the author who said that "the ultimate protection of both prisoners and investigators lies in the character of the review group, whose members are such as to insure detachment, expertise, fairness, and a sense of ethics."[3]

I would, therefore, offer this as an empirical study that responds with fifteen years of experience in a single setting to many of the anecdotes that have been implied as having complete generalization. I do not believe that the anecdotes are inappropriate or untrue, but to suggest that they represent universal conditions reflects ignorance of such an example as I have cited.

Once again, it seems to me that we have spent abundant time defining the dilemma; we should turn now to a synthesis that might offer a solution to the problem of maintaining the benefits of research while avoiding an exploitation of the prisoner.

INQUIRY AND COMMENTARY

LEWIS THOMAS: Before calling for comments and questions from the floor, I would like to take a few minutes for the members of the panel to turn to each other.

SABIN: Mr. Bronstein and I exchanged manuscripts for the first time yesterday. The ideas he expressed in it are ones that I would really like to have clarified. I am going to state your position, and then I would really like to be clear whether this is what we are arguing about.

First -- and this I got out of what you said this morning, although your manuscript says it another way -- the prison system in the United States is not capable of being reformed. Second, de facto environment of prisons is such that you *cannot* create -- my emphasis -- an institution in which informed consent without coercion is feasible. Prisons are inherently coercive, are not in any real sense rehabilitative, do not provide any real earning power, and are situated so as to involve maximum interference with the prisoner's life. And third, therefore if you cannot have consent without coercion, experimentation on prisoner subjects should not be permitted.

I would like to comment on these three points, and then ask you to give your position. You are not trying to convert me; I am not trying to convert you. We are trying to make a position clear.

BRONSTEIN: What you just said is my position.

SABIN: You agree then?

BRONSTEIN: Yes.

SABIN: So if I try to elucidate this, then I would like to say the following: that in my judgment, some of the bad situations you ascribe to the prison system did not prevail even twenty-two years ago in the Federal Reformatory at Chillicothe, Ohio, where I worked with several hundred prisoners over a period of three years. When I first came there I thought I was approaching a college campus, all the prisoners were working in industries. The Warden first had the idea of refusing me the freedom to do anything because it would destroy his industrial output. It was only after throwing the thing open to the prisoners, who are supposed to have no freedom of choice at all, that they consented to proceed with this without any increase in their pay or any other seduction than explaining to them the opportunity that they had of being of service.

Now if they had ulterior motives of perhaps getting their sentence shortened, I don't want to deprive them of that. If any parole board wishes to be influenced by, let us say, those prisoners who do elect to do that sort of thing and the 90 percent who do not, well that is up to the parole board. I don't want to deprive some prisoners of the opportunity to get this advantage.

Moreover, when you ask if research can be made to compensate for the barrenness of most of prison life by providing something to do, I want to say that this is not the purpose of medical research. It is not supposed to make up for it. It makes up a little. I don't want to deprive them of that.

Can medical research be used by the prison to cover the incompetence and the irrelevance of other prison programs? Certainly not, but that is a problem for the prisons. We are not here to argue the penal condition and the spectrum of prisons in the United States. I think we are here concerned only with the question of whether or not the good that comes to the prisoner who volunteers, and the good that comes to society as a result of experimentation under strict conditions of isolation and prolonged observation, should be abolished, and whether freedom of choice is completely absent in the prison to the extent that informed consent about the experiment is not feasible. The informed consent here is about the experiment that is to be done, not whether he should be restricted in body and so on while he is a prisoner to serve a sentence. Those are the issues.

BRONSTEIN: Let me try to respond a little, although I think I have probably answered or covered all of that in my presentation. I would like to raise one or two other things. Obviously I cannot speak about what happened in Chillicothe twenty years ago. Chillicothe is now a state institution -- it is not even a federal institution -- and is in fact a monstrosity.

Prison industries today in the federal system are total make-work. They have no rehabilitative quality. The General Accounting Office has been very critical of the whole federal prison industries program. I cannot believe that it is any worse today than it was twenty years ago.

I think the problem really is, Dr. Sabin, that you somehow have gotten the idea that as an advocate on behalf of prisoners, we are attempting to change, reform, eliminate the present prison system, using medical experimentation as the vehicle. That is not the case. Medical experimentation is just one small piece of the problem. It happens to be the piece we are discussing today. Our primary concern in the work we do throughout the country is not eliminating medical experimentation on human subjects in a captive situation. That is merely one manifestation of the problem of these institutions in our country.

I think, for example, to look at the case that Dr. Hubbard mentions, everything I said about prisons earlier applies, only more so, to the Michigan State Prison at Jackson. That prison is one of the most gross monstrosities in this country. There are no rehabilitative programs in that prison, any more than there are in any other prisons in this country. Mail is absolutely censored in and out of that institution. Our mail, labeled on the envelope in print, "This is attorney-client mail. Do not open except in the presence of the prisoner," is censored. Our mail is violated every day that we write to prisoners in Jackson. Their mail to us is censored as well.

The problem is that scientists really do not understand the nature of prisons. For Dr. Hubbard to stand up and talk about the rehabilitative quality and the recreational quality of this hundred-year-old, 4,400 man institution behind walls in Michigan, when most corrections people are condemning that institution in particular, and institutions like it, merely means that Dr. Hubbard does not understand the nature of that prison environment.

Let me go on to something that was mentioned by both of you because I think it is quite important. This motivation that you see, prisoners that feel that this is a way to rehabilitate themselves, and keep in mind that I did not say that prisoners should have no right to volunteer, what we are talking about is legal, informed consent based on the qualitative degree of intrusion that is involved in human experimentation.

Dr. Sabin directly, and Dr. Hubbard inferentially, referred to the recent Fordham-Yale Prison Research Project, which holds itself out as the first scientific study of prisoner motivation in human experimentation. The report was just released a month or two ago on the study.

First of all, there are some ethical questions about the study itself. The study was built on the big lie. These researchers, psychologists and psychiatrists, went into the Somers State Prison in Connecticut and told the prisoners that they represented a drug company, that they were really drug researchers, not psychological researchers, and represented that they were testing a new drug, whereas they were really testing the psychological motivation of prisoners.

Some interesting things came out of that study. For example, of the people tested, after two weeks of testing, 56 percent were unable to recall the intended uses of the drug, even though the testers claimed that they told them what the use was. After two weeks, 68 percent of the prisoners claimed that the drug had never previously been tested on human subjects, when the testers claimed that they told them it had. Now they decide that those remarkable statistics are because the prisoners really wanted to believe that; they blocked out the fact that they were told that there was prior testing. They really wanted to believe that so they could be martyrs, be heroes, feel that they were making a real contribution, and there is no scientific evidence to support that conclusion in this entire report.

The report concludes by saying, "First, research of diverse kinds, medical, clinical, psychological, social-psychological, sociological, experimental-psychological, and in fact, any research meeting fundamental criteria of non-aversiveness, non-intrusiveness, practicability, and meaningfulness should be incorporated within the program structure of the institution as a significant component of the rehabilitation and image management system."

That is precisely the kind of abuse I was trying to refer to before. These scientists -- these happen not to be medical scientists, but psychiatrists -- believe that anything can be done. They take the position that anything goes as long as -- and they set out these things that are not possible -- it's nonaversive, nonintrusive, practicable, meaningful, and should be a significant component of the image management and rehabilitation program.

Let me tell you what one prisoner who participated in that wrote us, to give you an idea of the kind of con job, if you will, that you have been subjected to. This is a prisoner participating in this study:

> Not many prisoners get physically screwed up on these tests. The reason: we do not take the drug. When blood-drawing is due, we take a small piece of the pill, but the rest is not taken. Out of a thirty-man test, they may get five or six fools to take it as they hand it out.
> When they were drawing blood and taking urine samples, I never took any but a couple of chips during the whole test,

and many did likewise. This has to show when twenty to twenty-five guys are doing it out of thirty. Also the few fools who were taking the shit, I and others had piss in the containers when possible for us, plus theirs. Plus if I would give my No. 25 test tube for blood to someone taking the drug, then I would grab his, erase the number on it, put my 25 on it after he was drawn for blood.

But this test is money, not the humantarian aspects of drug testing. After all, all agreed to participate even before they knew the money was funded. They also let it leak out that if this test if not conducted, we will have no other test ever, and that the $30,000 lost to prisoners since Pfizer was shut down will be lost forever. Many, many prisoners want that money, and they will agree to any damn thing to get the big $200 and $300 tests back in here.

That is the motivation.

SABIN: I challenge it. It says one minor sample is incorrect from beginning to end for the total picture.

HUBBARD: Mr. Bronstein is a very skillful advocate, and of course one of the classical ploys is to discredit the witness if you cannot debate his actual statements.

The fact of the matter is that I am very familiar with the system in Michigan, having served as Chairman of the Governor's Correction Commission for over two years, and having made in-depth visits, including free and untrammeled interviews with prisoners in all of the major institutions in that state.

Mr. Bronstein said that there are no rehabilitation programs at the Jackson prison. This is either a euphemistic expression of the general recognition of failure of success of rehabilitation, or a gross misstatement of fact. I assume that it was the former.

He has also mentioned that his mail was censored. I would ask that he document that, and if this is the case I will see that disciplinary action is taken for those involved. The fact is as I stated it, and this is part of the law of the state of Michigan.

The problem then is not to lay anecdote on anecdote, but to ask oneself whether this dilemma has a synthesis available. And I would urge again that we examine this case that I have presented, not as a contest of whether one wandering medical scientist knows what he is talking about, but from the record and from the future that we have to contend with.

FRANCIS D. MOORE: I am from the Harvard Medical School. I would like to change the subject from drug testing to scarce anatomical resources. In the early days of kidney transplantation, prisoners were permitted to volunteer for a kidney donation, and in one unit in this country several transplants were done on that basis. Before

143

the advent of tissue typing and cross-matching, there was a clear advantage to the living donor over the cadaver donor, and there still is. However, my own feeling was that there was an element of coercion here, no matter how subtle, for a person to undertake a surgical operation that permanently altered his body and his future potential for injury, especially if he were again involved in a violent crime of any sort. So mainly because of my own distaste for this, it was stopped completely.

In our own state, a prisoner was condemned to death, and the date of his execution was set prior to the Supreme Court decision. I am happy to say it was never carried out. But in anticipation of his execution, he and his family offered to donate several of his organs for transplantation. It so turned out that his blood type was compatible with a patient who had been waiting for three years for a kidney. We never did do a tissue typing on him. I felt that there was a tiny element here, however small, in the balance of decision as to pardon or commutation of the sentence. My own decision was therefore strongly negative, and we with thanks and gratitude refused to use his organs had he been executed.

I would therefore like to ask the panel what they would have done, or what they perceive as appropriate for organ donation on a voluntary basis from prisoners, or assignment of organs from individuals executed for crime.

THOMAS: Could I ask the panel to file that away along with the other matters that will turn up, rather than interrupt, because I would like to work our way back through the hall.

STUART BROWN: I am affiliated with the Science, Technology and Society program at Cornell University. I am a philosopher, and it is as a philosopher that I want to speak. I find Bronstein's argument flawless. Like all flawless arguments, I suppose it depends upon the premises. Dr. Hubbard said something that was intended to weaken that premise, and I want to try to correct that.

What Dr. Hubbard said is that there is a logical positivist doctrine that all human actions are caused, and that if we accept this, it somehow or other removes the difference between coerced and uncoerced actions. The first thing is that the doctrine that all human actions are caused is centuries old. It is an old Christian doctrine that was held by people like St. Augustine.

The second thing is that Jonathan Edwards, in a beautiful piece on that subject, showed with flawless, logical argument that even if you hold it, it does not remove the moral and logical difference between coerced and uncoerced actions.

ROBERT BURT: I am from the University of Michigan Law School. I would like to suggest and hear the panel's reaction to a shift in focus on the way that we might approach this problem.

If one looks at the issue, it seems to me, of consent in its own terms, the argument can go on forever and ever, and very closely

144

joined. On the one hand, it is crystal clear that the coercions are enormous within a prison setting; but on the other hand, one can always argue that they may be equivalent to lots of coercion on lots of different people, the dying as one instance, that are not used as sufficient grounds to rule out an entire population as experimental subjects.

And then there is the other argument that went back and forth -- what better protects the dignity of those people, to withhold choice from them, or indeed to give them a sense of choice within all of the other constraints? It seems to me that that argument is a very difficult one to resolve.

But let me suggest a difference in focus. It seems to me that the underlying problem here and the underlying risk that we are grappling with is the danger that in the course of medical experimentation we identify some parts of the population as less than human, as special targets for dehumanizing kinds of things. That, in turn, has all kinds of unhealthy multiplier effects, and there is a very special danger with the groups we talked about yesterday -- fetuses, children -- and with the group that will be talked about later today, and prisoners are importantly among those.

Well, if that is the special danger, as I think it is, it seems to me that a solution, a beginning of the solution to that, would be to insist on, in all cases possible, and perhaps even as a blanket rule, an equivalent treatment for experimental purposes for those who are in prisons and those who are out of prisons as one way of insisting that we are not targeting these people especially. In essence, what I am suggesting is for general research protocols to insist that there be the same research protocol carried out in the free community as inside a prison population, as one of the grounds for letting it go forward.

There are practical difficulties with that. Let me just address two of them. One, the problem of finding a long-term sequestered population. Yes, of course, they are available in prisons. But there are other places in this society where we do manage to find long-term sequestered populations for what are perceived to be socially-important purposes. One example that I can think of is the Watergate jury -- a highly motivated group that saw the social significance of what they were doing and were willing to give up a lot for the virtues of this.

It seems to me, then, that if we are serious about the proposition we are not dehumanizing, we would be willing to set up research protocols that make it worthwhile for extra-prison populations. But there is yet another difficulty, and that is the point that Mr. Bronstein very nicely made: How reliable is the research that goes on inside these institutions because of the feeling and the way that these prisoners conduct themselves?

What you really echo, it seems to me, is the analysis that Richard Titmuss made in his lovely book, *The Gift Relationship*, in

which he talks about what the commercialization of blood donations
in this country, in fact, does to the worth of those blood donations,
and how the motive that brings people forward means that we have an
enormous problem of hepatitis, an enormous problem of donors playing
games and lying, as compared to the English situation as he suggests.

It seems to me that this would then suggest that it is vitally
important to have a free population control group in order to make
sure that you don't have artifice coming from the motivations of
prisoners inside.

So there are at least two reasons for such a proposal. First for
research on its own terms and the value to it of having a free population. Second, even more importantly, to see to it that we are not
targeting a group for dehumanization, which does terrible things to
all of us.

STUART SPICKER: I don't think we should, after today, rest complacent
with the formulation of the basic arguments along an empirical
spectrum. Dr. Hubbard honestly presented it that way, and that is
what we have heard. There are other kinds of arguments, not empirical. By empirical I mean the longer or the better institutions get
at preserving certain kinds of environments within, the more we are
justified in intervening by having subjects of experimentation who
are prisoners. That is the empirical procedure that we have heard.

There is also a more fundamental kind of approach, but not as
clear and easy to deal with as the empirical, namely, that the autonomy of prisoners is, in principal, violated. They are prisoners;
they are not free. I don't know how we can turn that around, I don't
care how good the penal system.

So you can take the argument to say the empirical determinants
are totally irrelevant. The autonomy of these individuals is in
fact undercut, and therefore a whole new set of arguments may follow.

The second point is related to that. Even if X gives his or her
informed consent, as it has been defined so far, and it is a very
muddled term, it does not follow at all that we, outside such an
institution with incarcerated human beings, have a right to even
make the request.

GEORGE HILL: My question is directed to Dr. Hubbard. We don't often
get a president in front of us to decide for us the rights and wrongs
of a particular situation in which he has been involved for fifteen
years.

There is a question there on the floor as to the validity not only
of the research, but of the actual prisoners' conditions as described
by the president of this gigantic corporation. I would like to ask
him a question or two directly in this procedure.

What are the profits that the company and the corporation has
made in these fifteen years of research in that institution at
Jackson? Has the corporation used any of its funds to better the
condition of the prisoners in that facility? And, may I ask, is

146

this corporation willing to set up a fund if the state organizations
are not prepared to pay living wages, or minimum wages, under federal guidelines? Would you care to offer a fund for prisoners'
advancement as human beings, as well as guinea pigs?

HUBBARD: I have no way of knowing what the commercial value has been;
these are very early experiments, most of which never result in a
product that sees the market.

HILL: May I ask how much money you have invested in this losing proposition?

HUBBARD: Our research runs at about $55 to $60 million a year.

HILL: Do you write that off as a tax deduction, as a loss?

HUBBARD: No. That is an ordinary business expense.

HILL: Do your stockholders know exactly what the results of those
fifteen years of careful research have brought the company?

HUBBARD: I am not sure whether we are in a dialogue or I am answering
some questions.

HILL: We are in both.

HUBBARD: Yes, all of the results of our research are published both in
the scientific literature and in the lay literature.

UNIDENTIFIED: I have a remark and a question directed to Dr. Sabin.
During my residency, several of my colleagues moonlighted at the
correctional institution at Chillicothe. They made several compari-
sons of the institution to various things, and I don't recall that a
college campus was one of them. The only thing I can conclude is
that either college campuses have changed a lot, or else the institution has become a lot more refreshing.
    Studies on patient satisfaction and dissatisfaction with health
care services have often turned up findings that were surprising to
the physicians involved in their care. When interviewed by people
not identified with the health care institutions, patients often
expressed dissatsifaction that they do not express to their
physicians. This is not particularly surprising, given the asymmetry
of the physician-patient relationship and the resulting reluctance
of patients to criticize their doctors face to face.
    Another reason for physicians not being aware of their patients'
dissatisfactions is the phenomenon called selective perception. This
phenomenon is also not surprising, since most people are not capable
of rigorous self-examination and not especially sensitive to

criticisms of their behavior that are particularly subtle, and sometimes even if they are overt.

I think that these phenomena occur with clinical investigation and with investigators trying to evaluate their own research. I am delighted that your volunteers all expressed altruistic motivations for their volunteering, and I am also delighted that you seem to have overcome the problems with selective perception and with patients' reluctance to criticize.

My question is, how did you do it? I think that really could be of benefit to a lot of us here.

THOMAS: We have one more question.

RICHARD WADE: I am Director of Program Services for the American Public Health Association. I have two points, and then one recommendation.

First of all, I do disagree with Drs. Hubbard and Sabin in that coercion is minimal, and I lean on the side of Mr. Bronstein.

After considerable debate over the last several years, the American Public Health Association has taken a stand, siding with Mr. Bronstein in terms of coercion in prisons, that it is suitable to call for a reduction or elimination of biomedical research in prisons.

My recommendation is that until state and national policies are developed for putting greater constraints on research in prisons, those people who serve on institutional review committees should ask two questions: Why and So what? Why are prisoners being used? And what are the consequences of not using prisoners? If these kinds of questions are asked of each individual researcher and protocol, then we might find that prisoners have in fact been used because they are convenient and accessible, and that exploitation really has and continues to go on.

WILLIAM SMITH: I am with the Children's Defense Fund, and I have a couple of questions for Dr. Hubbard. Yesterday there were many references to a climate of openness. You have described the fact that the Upjohn Company conducts experiments on prisoners in Jackson, Michigan. I would like to know whether your company sponsors, or whether your scientists do drug testing on incarcerated juvenile delinquents.

HUBBARD: Not to my knowledge. We do, however, do research on a volunteer group from an open community with the same protocols essentially that are used in Jackson.

SMITH: These are children in Jackson?

HUBBARD: No, no. Jackson has no children.

SMITH: Do you do drug testing on children?

HUBBARD: Generally not, because the conditions for drug testing in pediatrics are now so constraining that in effect one does not have the opportunity available.

SMITH: So your drugs are not tested on children?

HUBBARD: They are not utilized in children.

SMITH: No Upjohn Company drug is utilized for a child?

HUBBARD: The majority of our drugs have not gone through testing with children, and this is true of all pharmaceutical companies. We have some drugs that have. Pediatric formulation of our antibiotics, of course, has been tested in children. But the conditions of testing of antibiotics are a special case and not typical of the regulations for testing of all other therapeutic entities. The simple fact of the matter is that the constraints on drug testing in pediatrics today has created a very serious problem in maintaining a flow of new therapeutic agents into the hands of pediatricians. This is true not only of our company, but of all companies.

THOMAS: I would like to ask the panel now to finish. Dr. Sabin, do you want to put in some concluding remarks?

SABIN: Yes. I think first of all, going backwards, a reply is needed for the record to Dr. Wade from the American Public Health Association. I agree with him that we must always give a good reason why a particular piece of research should be done in a prison and not elsewhere.

There is a great deal of research going on outside of prisons. Now the reason for doing something in a prison is first of all to prevent, let's say with an infectious disease like malaria, infecting the community at large. There also is the possibility of follow-up. Prisoners are captive only in the sense that society has made them captive, and therefore they are useful for long follow-up. Whereas, if you get somebody from the outside and you pay him $20 a day -- that is also being done -- three months from now he is off on some other project.

So there are special conditions and situations that make prisons especially useful settings that cannot easily be duplicated outside.

The next important question that he posed is what would be the consequences if, for whatever minimal reasons, we agreed completely with the conclusion of Mr. Bronstein that all experiments should be stopped in prisons. What would happen to medical research?

I would say that it would be greatly impeded. We would have to recruit populations as people are recruited for armies, put them under conditions of isolation, be able to keep them for a number of years and follow them. We are spending money for lots of other things. I don't care about the money, but then we would have other scruples. Who would apply for a job like that? He would be unemployed, he would be mentally disturbed. He would have all sorts of other things that coerce him into participating in something like that. So the consequences of not doing it would be a tremendous impediment to the type of research that can be done only in prisons.

Now I would like to go back to the college campus idea, and also to the business of the letter that my good friend, Mr. Bronstein, read. We are dealing in all of these things with spectra. One person is part, one point on a spectrum; one college campus at one end of the spectrum may be much worse than some of the prisons. The point is that we are dealing with a complex situation, and not with any one point on the spectrum. Therefore, the real issue is this: whether as a result of all these considerations the only conclusion is that you have got to shut off all prison populations from the opportunity for volunteering -- and even though it does not really rehabilitate them to the extent that one would like, it is an opportunity to somehow or other modify their lives, and I think beneficially; or whether we continue as we are, but under the greatest safeguards, and only for the most important things, and to comply with the specific requirements as were stated before by the American Public Health Association.

BRONSTEIN: In answer to the questions from the floor: I would take the same position with respect to the contribution of organs that Dr. Moore took. Everyone else, as far as I can tell, either agreed substantially or entirely with everything I had to say, so there is no point in commenting.

As far as the question of where do we get this population for testing if we do not use prisoners, I would suggest that all middle- and top-level executives of the twenty largest drug companies and their families would be the ideal populations.

THOMAS: Dr. Hubbard, do you want to have a last word?

HUBBARD: I will just remark that for someone who is interested in non-coercive consent, that is a remarkable suggestion.

THE POOR

Franz J. Ingelfinger
Henry W. Foster
Jay Katz

FRANZ INGELFINGER

To define *the poor*, one might use the purely economic criterion. Or,
from what we have heard in this Forum, one might argue that anyone who
is a subject of human experimentation is poor -- that is, poor like a
guinea pig. But our definition is intermediate. We shall use *poor* to
encompass those populations that are deprived not only for strictly economic reasons, but because of social, cultural, administrative, and political factors.

Each of us will discuss selected major issues pertaining to the use
of the poor for experimental purposes. Since the poor have been disproportionately used for experimentation -- and each of us agrees on
this point -- specific illustrative cases are not short in supply.
Indeed, some of the most notorious cases of human exploitation for research have involved the poor.

My two colleagues are particularly conversant with one of these, the
so-called Tuskegee Study on the natural history of syphilis. Dr. Katz
was a member of the Ad Hoc Advisory Panel established by HEW to investigate this study. Dr. Foster was President of the County Medical Society
in the area where the study was carried out at the time that news of it
broke. I have had no such firsthand experience. However, I am not prepared to take, in the interest of fomenting controversy, the position
that the poor are ideal experimental, sacrificial subjects.

Our objectives in this discussion are: to assess if the poor now are,
and will continue to be, particularly exposed to use, abuse, or both as
subjects of human experimentation; to examine the reasons why the poor
may be more likely to be used or abused as experimental subjects; and

to explore means that could be devised to ensure that the assumption of risk by the poor does not exceed that of the rest of the population.

HENRY FOSTER

After I had agreed to participate on this panel, I felt that I could make my most worthwhile contribution, and indeed help create the Forum atmosphere, by raising an issue that had at least three components. First, I wanted to bring an issue that had some reasonable degree of feasibility to it. Second, I wanted to bring an issue that would not be agreed upon by at least one, or maybe both, of my panel colleagues. And third, I wanted to raise an issue that would not likely be otherwise raised. I think I may have been successful in the latter two.

In searching for solutions to the special problems resulting from human experimentation in the poor, their exemption from such participation, in my judgment, warrants strong consideration. In the course of my deliberations, however, it is essential to keep in mind that the concepts put forth here on this issue of such prodigious complexity are directed not to the whole of the biomedical research pool, but only to a small segment. As a physician who is also directly involved in academia, I am left with the feeling of some ambivalence following my recommendation.

In spite of the many shortcomings in the realm of human experimentation, it must be emphasized that this country's biomedical research community has been a world leader in its concern for medical ethics. As recently as 1960, no articles on this subject except in the English language could be found in the world literature. However, in spite of this concern, the thalidomide disaster and subsequent events set into motion a greater public demand for control. This demand in this country is expressed in the popular movement known as consumerism and, specifically, in that movement's concern with the right to know.

In the biomedical research community, it is expressed in the requirement for voluntary informed consent-giving on the part of patients. Given such universal concern, any perverse outcomes in research in humans today would indeed be most inopportune, especially if such research design were characterized by demonstrable disruption of the balance between risks and benefits for the patient. Parenthetically, recent untoward outcomes of this nature are in great part responsible for our being assembled here today.

In this day of heightened consumer awareness, occurrences such as the Tuskegee syphylis experiment, the injection of cancer cells into uninformed geriatric patients, and the deception of Chicano women seeking contraception cannot and will not be allowed to continue in this country. Although such cases are by far the exception, they are nonetheless very likely to be viewed by consumers as the rule. The call to consider a moratorium on the use of the poor in human experimentation thus stems as much from pragmatism as it does from altruism.

152

Indispensable to ethical biomedical research is the balance of two values: scientific priority of discovery, on the one hand; and humane therapeutic treatment, on the other. This has come to be known as the dilemma of science and therapy. There are those who fear for the scientific priority if there is a shift in this equation from its current status, and to exempt the poor, even temporarily, from human experimentation would create such a threat to research in the minds of some. However, if properly structured, such a moratorium would not be a hindrance; failure on the part of the biomedical sector to take such a step will have far graver consequences for both scientific and public interests and values. This alteration in policy should be intrinsic, and if the biomedical community fails to do so, we can be assured of increased hostility and of public demand for even more external control.

By some estimates it is believed that possibly 80 percent of all human experimentation that has occurred in this country involved the poor. How then can it be plausible to waive the participation of this group? The answer, in part, relates to the makeup of the group normally characterized as the poor. Although implicit in the term *poor*, as stated in my colleague's introductory remarks, it is the social and cultural deprivation that is of primary significance as it relates to this whole question, rather than the lack of economic resources per se. There are many who are classified as poor who do not suffer deep and grinding social and cultural deprivation, and therefore need not be considered for exemption.

How then is it to be determined who is so deprived, and thus subject to exemption from human experimentation? It is my belief that those incapable of clearly providing voluntary informed consent constitute this group. They are the functionally illiterate, the senile, those who do not command the English language, and certainly the mentally incompetent.

Irrespective of the definition one chooses to use, however, it is apparent that the biomedical sector has come to rely too heavily and in a disproportionate fashion on the use of the poor for human research. We should be reminded that the poor constitute a relatively small proportion of this nation's total population. Moreover, we should begin to look beyond the poor for human research subjects, with the ultimate expectation that this segment of our population will dwindle.

According to the Bureau of Statistics, there were just over 24 million persons in this country classified as below low-income levels in March of 1973. Even if this number were doubled, there would still remain more than 150 million nonpoor who would be, and in fact have become, more accessible to research usage as the mode of health care financing changes -- an issue with implications of its own.

What should we hope to accomplish during the suggested moratorium? This interim should be used to reexamine those factors that tend to disrupt that balance between science and therapy, and thus restructure those mechanisms necessary to maintain that equilibrium that spawns the most favorable milieu for both humane values and scientific priority.

As with any socially structured system, conflicts develop in the application of values by those who are part of the system, resulting in compliant and deviant behavior. There are social control processes that when operative tend to preclude deviant behavior. These processes take the form of socialization or training, collaboration groups and informal networks, and forms of peer review. There is a great need for the socialization of human values in medical school and beyond, as has been pointed out so well by Renée Fox.

Studies show that the socialization of scientific values is well ahead of that of human values. Characteristics of collaboration groups and informal networks that lend to deviant behavior could possibly be improved if changes were made in the process of academic reward and advancement and in the financing of medical education. Although external pressures for peer review continue to be applied, there remain other refinements and innovations that can, and ought to, originate from within our ranks.

In conclusion, I must reiterate that our profession today is under the greatest scrutiny ever, and it behooves us to consider the measures mentioned in this presentation -- measures that should help to prevent new human catastrophes. Further disasters at this juncture will do far greater harm to the interests of biomedical research than will the exemption of a small, vulnerable segment of our population.

JAY KATZ

Should what I have to say sound like a communication from Mars, I would like to apologize beforehand.

Human experimentation can be hazardous to its subjects. Thus it is not surprising that the economically and socially disadvantaged are conscripted for research to a disproportionately large extent. Throughout histroy the poor have been indentured for society's most disagreeable tasks, and medical science has only followed time-honored patterns of recruitment.

It may seem regrettable that in the name of progress, science too requires its unwilling subjects. Yet for the benefit of present and future generations, science and society have always tolerated human sacrifices: the Aztec gods demanded them lest the universe fall apart; the fires of the Inquisition consumed them lest faith be diminished; and Apollo, the Physician, permitted them lest disease not be understood and conquered.

It would be an exercise in futility to curb tradition by focusing merely on the poor and insulating them from participation in research. Such a limited objective would only create new groups of cheap bodies who are not unidentifiable by a means test. If today's or tomorrow's poor are to benefit from our concern over their fate, we must not surround them with special safeguards, but rather look to the underlying causes that make the poor particularly, though not solely, vulnerable to exploitation in research.

Those who advocate special protection for the poor have argued that the poor cannot comprehend what participation in research requires of them, and that they are inherently vulnerable to external coercions. To be sure, subjects will be found among the poor, perhaps more than in the population at large, who cannot understand what is being asked of them and they, like all incompetents, should not be allowed to participate except under unusual and well-defined circumstances. But many will remain who do understand. Comprehension is not the problem; at least it is not a greater problem with the poor than with other research participants.

With respect to coercions, we must distinguish between those created by persons' life situations, and those imposed by the interpersonal dynamics of investigators and their subjects. Life situations, be they poverty or physical disability, have an impact on all persons. But these conditions, however unequal, together with persons' inner dynamics, define what human beings are and, at the time of decision, can be. We may wish to approach persons who live in particularly unfortunate social circumstances with greater care to make sure that we do not further reduce, through deliberate acts of our own, the more limited range of alternatives available to them. But beyond that, we must honor their decisions as much as we should those of persons more affluently situated.

It is equally demeaning to assert that persons' consent should be rejected because if they were wiser or more rational they would have made different decisions, as it is to assert that their consent should not be trusted because if they only were richer they would have chosen differently. Ultimately, we must bow to the best decisions persons can make as they are situated. And we must accept their decisions in the firm belief that every human being knows his own world better than any outsider, even if the outsider is a physician or an investigator.

The notion that the poor have an impaired capacity to comprehend or by virtue of their external life situations cannot make their own decisions is a stereotypical and degrading view of them. It is the coercion resulting from physician-investigators' interpersonal interactions with the poor that create more serious problems. Here too we know that such coercions are not necessarily restricted to interactions with poor subjects. If they create special problems for them, we must look for other reasons.

I believe that the problems with the poor, as well as with all subjects of experimentation, originate in an insufficiently analyzed conflict of values inherent in the conduct of human research: the quest for the acquisition of knowledge for the benefit of present and future generations on the one hand; and respect for the dignity, autonomy, and inviolability (unless consented to) of the subjects of research. I am not addressing here only or even primarily the issue of harm to subjects, but rather the question so succinctly raised by Isaiah Berlin: "In the name of what can [we] ever be justified in forcing men to do what they have not willed or consented to?" I do not wish to suggest that this value conflict is very frequently as abysmally weighted in favor of "progress" as, for example, in the Tuskegee syphilis study, the Nazi concentration camp experiments, or the countless venereal disease studies perpetrated all over the world in the late nineteenth and twentieth centuries. However, I do wish to suggest that in balancing the two conflicting values, the research community has generally not only come out in favor of the acquisition of knowledge but also neglected to confront consciously the consequences of such a choice.

Pious exhortation calling for respect of the subjects of research or mindless risk-benefit formulae have not served us well as decisional guides. The contraceptive studies with Chicano women are cases in point. Is it permissible to give them placebo-contraceptives without informing them, and then to add insult to injury by not providing them with the opportunity for abortion because state laws prohibit them? This also is true of the various randomization studies in which patient-subjects are told that they will be assigned to different treatment groups on the basis of their medical needs, while in fact they are assigned by lot. All these studies are justified by the need to advance medical knowledge so that future patients will not be condemned to the fate of "therapeutic orphans" for lack of research data.

I do not question the need for controlled clinical trials in the humane practice of medicine; I only wish to question the thoughtlessness about the rights of the subjects with which many of these trials are being conducted. Once the balancing process is tilted in favor of science and society and against the individual, and the choice is made without asking why, when, and at what cost -- why particularly seems such an unnecessary question -- the rest follows easily. Then subjects must be found, then "unavoidable" shortcuts can be taken in the name of the higher value. The other value, respect for the individual, can in turn be neglected. Thus, the subjects of research have found themselves on the slippery slope of exploitation without any clear answer to the question: When, if ever, are exploitation, deceit, and misrepresentation warranted?

At the same time, of course, investigators are not unaffected by this value choice because in its consequences to subjects it goes counter to some of their human feelings. However, there exists, I believe, in investigators an enormous ambivalence toward the subjects of research, reflected in conflicting wishes to care and to reject, to treat and to mistreat, to protect and to destroy, to elevate and to degrade. Such ambivalence is deeply rooted in the character structure of many persons who become investigators, and it is an expression of the tensions created by viewing their subjects both as fellow human beings and as objects of research. Such ambivalence has blinded them to their tampering, via the balancing of values in favor of science, with fundamental principles of respect for the individual -- principles that in theory, but not necessarily in practice, are dear to society as well as to medicine.

Sorting out this value conflict cannot be left to the individual conscience of investigators. It requires, first of all, a relentless confrontation of the consequences that a balancing of values in favor of

156

science and society and against the individual subject would entail, and then a determination of how far the neglect of either value should be permitted to proceed. Once such an analysis has been undertaken, investigators will at least have the opportunity to compare their practices against some kind of an external standard. The plea to leave this determination to the investigator's conscience is an expression of science's and society's readiness to keep sufficiently ambiguous the consequences of contemporary research practices and even to encourage investigators to neglect the individual in the interest of societal benefits, but to do so quietly and surreptitiously.

Respect for individual autonomy requires that one begin with total disclosure: sharing knowledge and admitting uncertainty and ignorance, answering all questions and identifying unanswerable ones, appreciating doubts and respecting fears. Such an obligation to disclose, a requisite of a genuine invitation, becomes an awesome encounter for the investigator if engaged in honestly. Consider what must be disclosed if it is taken seriously! Investigators' dread to engage in such a searching and explicit dialogue can remain unacknowledged by the rationalization that the demands of science require nondisclosure, and the preferred value supports such a decision.

Also in turning to research subjects from lower social classes, the reluctance to disclose is further rationalized by the unwarranted belief that the poor do not understand anyway. Why bother to explain? Is not the willingness of investigators to assume the heavy burden of becoming the guarantors of subjects' safety proof of their great responsibility toward them?

The preferred choice of the poor has other roots as well. Investigators, who generally come from higher social classes, have an impaired capacity to identify with the poor. This psychosocial fact contributes greatly to the ease with which the poor are chosen for participation in research, though a problem amenable to correction. For if we wished to take greater care in obtaining a more representative sample of the population for research purposes, we could do so. Computer technology has given us the tools to accomplish that objective.

Finally, in the pursuit of scientific progress, it is easy to overlook that progress is hard to define in general, and the gain to science from individual research projects difficult to predict in particular. In the light of these uncertainties, personal motivations, be they curiosity, fame, or professional advancement, can readily lead to an exaggerated estimate of the value of a research project to science. While there is nothing wrong with such motivations, they tend, unless care is taken, to subtly undermine investigators' respect for the subjects of research.

What lessons can be learned from the poor of research? Precious little that applies only to the poor once we have acknowledged that they have been used too exclusively and too uninformedly. Even the problems created by lack of disclosure extend beyond the poor to other research participants as well. Yet we could learn a lot if we viewed the treatment of the poor in research as telling evidence of problems inherent in contemporary research practices. What can be done?

(1) The conflicting values -- acquisition of knowledge and respect for the autonomy of the individual -- should be more openly acknowledged and subjected to a relentless scholarly and public scrutiny. I appreciate that the implementation of such a recommendation may create new tensions, for it would reveal that our commitment to life may not be very strong whenever it costs too much or whenever it interferes with other collective benefits we wish to obtain. Life is not a pearl beyond price; at least it has not been so up to now. It may prove too anxiety-provoking to bring this fact out into the open, particularly in the arena of medical research where patients are so frequently employed as subjects. Thus, since research must and will go forward, it has been argued that the mental health of society may be better served by avoiding the promulgation of clear and purposive choices as to whom to harm (without their consent) for the collective good. I submit that we take for once a different approach and try to decide more consciously and self-consciously whom we wish to use in medical research, under what circumstances, and with what safeguards.

(2) Our value priorities should be reordered in favor of total fidelity to the subjects of research. It may slow down research, impede the acquisition of knowledge and the advancement of science. Yet, might not future generations benefit more from an experiment that for once gave the highest priority to respect for the individuals who are living today and not tomorrow? After all, what is progress? Does it not point into many directions which we cannot pursue all at once and all at the same pace?

(3) We should insist that investigators sit down and talk with their prospective subjects as long as it takes, and until they are certain that the subjects understand what is being asked of them. Only those who do understand should be allowed to participate in research.

Last month we paid a small sum of money to the survivors of the Tuskegee syphilis study. Yet the best reparation we could pay them, as well as the poor of all ages, is to find answers to one question: What can we learn from our treatment of the poor that will improve the lot of all subjects of research? After all, the treatment of the disadvantaged has often been an indicator of the health of society. The health of science may also be reflected in how it treats its poor.

FRANZ INGELFINGER

My colleagues have alluded to some of the reasons why experimenters may have been inclined to use the poor as subjects. In particular, they have emphasized characteristics of the poor as individuals: the cultural, social, and educational deprivations that may make each poor person a more tractable subject. I should like to emphasize another feature that has made the poor desirable subjects for medical

158

investigation: the poor *as a group* have been administratively more eligible than other segments of the population.

By and large, the poor have received institutionalized care -- on
charity hospital wards, in the city hospital outpatient clinics, or as
charges of the Public Health Service. Thus, groups of the poor could
be more effectively divided, treated, and followed. Standardized and
unvarying regimens could be administered, and a consistent record for-
mat could be applied. The poor, if dissatisfied with their care, were
hardly in a position to change doctors. In particular, the poor lack
that hindrance to the investigator, that is, the private doctor who, to
be sure, might be profiting from a fee-for-service arrangement, but who
at the same time was independent enough to disrupt any efforts to stan-
dardize management, who was erratic enough to keep heterogenous and
often undecipherable records, and who, above all, was ready to act as
an advocate for his paying patients.

(Dr. Thomas may remember that when we were in medical school we were
given a lecture on the care of a patient by one of Boston's most successful practitioners. Unfortunately, this otherwise imposing man
stuttered a bit. So, we were told that we must always keep in mind the
human needs of the pa-pa-pay-patient.)

The administrative eligibility of poor groups, that is, their regi-
mentability and their manageability as groups of experimental subjects,
deserves consideration for two reasons. In the first place, experimental use of the poor because of their administrative eligibility continues up to the present with, ironically enough, little opposition
from the parties very much concerned with the rights and dignity of
much smaller groups of experimental subjects. Second, the number of
administratively eligible is steadily increasing and may eventually
include much of the population, present company not excepted. An example of use of the poor because of their administrative eligibility is
provided by recent studies involving over a million of California's
economically deprived, the so-called Medi-Cal beneficiaries.

In 1970, a trial was instituted to determine whether hospitalization
for Medi-Cal patients could be decreased by a state-enforced requirement that all nonemergency Medi-Cal admissions must be approved for
hospital admission and for a specific number of days of stay, such
approval being obligatory before admission. Results: as compared to
numbers expected on the basis of previous experience, days of hospitalization for the poor during a nine-month period were reduced by about
16 percent. In a similar trial, run under somewhat different auspices,
a 17-percent decrease in days of hospital utilization was achieved.

The results of these studies were acclaimed as evidence that hospital
overutilization could be contained. But, to the best of my knowledge,
there was no way of telling whether the hospital days saved were merely
at the expense of overutilization or whether, indeed, the health of the
poor had been adversely affected.

In another experiment, in 1971-72, nearly a million Medi-Cal beneficiaries were placed on co-payment status, that is, they had to pay
one dollar for the first of two medical visits each month and fifty

cents for each of the first two prescriptions each month. Those who conducted the study decided that the co-pay features did not interfere with the care of what they called serious illness. Yet, in the Aid for Dependent Children program, co-payers obtained immunizations at about half the rate of non-co-payers, and 9 percent of the AFDC group reported that co-payment had deterred them from seeking medical care.

In the experiments just cited the immediate goal was not hygienic but economic discovery: Could the poor be taken care of more cheaply? But obviously hospitalization was withheld from the poor rather than other segments of the population because the Medi-Cal population and its records could be more readily controlled and effectively analyzed. Similar use of many whose health care is supported by state or federal government is far from unimaginable should a need be perceived for other socioeconomic medical experiments related to health care or for randomized clinical trials on the effectiveness of a certain prophylactic health measure.

If the poor will continue to attract investigators because of their administrative eligibility, one may ask who are these poor? Are Veterans Administration patients, because they receive institutional and governmental care, poor? Since they are also administratively eligible -- even more so than the economically poor -- they might be called socially deprived, and hence, according to this panel's definition, poor. Thus, most large-scale randomized clinical trials these days, it should be realized, whether of drugs for hypertension, cancer management, or surgical procedures, are the results of cooperative VA studies.

In the future, depending on what type of national health insurance is promulgated, perhaps most of us will be "poor" in the sense that we will acquire the characteristics of administrative eligibility: easily accessible and standardized records, manageability, and susceptibility to follow-up control. In the United Kingdom, for example, randomized clinical trials appear to have been carried out more effectively and more frequently than here. A number of explanations may be offered, but one is the administrative availability of the population under the National Health Service. In spite of Dr. McDermott's comments yesterday, we are now in the heyday of the randomized trial, and conduct of that trial depends upon the conscription of large bodies of the population.

The expanding number of the poor as defined by us will benefit the economically poor, for their up-to-now particular burden will be distributed across much of the population. But much of the population -- and this is what concerns me -- may well be politically dominant, and such a majority, if its fears of becoming guinea pigs are accentuated, or if its attitudes are those as expressed by some of the members of the last panel yesterday, such fears may produce disastrous restraints or encumbrances on essential clinical investigation.

Present as well as future generations argue for the establishment of mechanisms that will protect administratively eligible groups from improper experimental procedure. The sizable if yet limited number of poor groups that exist today requires that protection for their sake. In the future the protection of the many more who will receive institutionalized or at least federally supervised care is necessary, I think, not only for their sake, but also for the sake of unstifled medical research.

INQUIRY AND COMMENTARY

GERARD PIEL: I am a publisher. But I speak now in all due diffidence as a philosopher. There has run through the contributions to this Forum, especially from those who are concerned with the urgency and the need of human subjects for medical research, the proposition that we are engaged in the balancing of values. The title of this session of the Forum is "Individual Risks Versus Societal Benefits." There is the notion that it is possible to balance the compromising of individual privacy and integrity on the one hand versus the need of society for the urgent tasks of medical research on the other. This has a kind of an American pragmatic sound about it. It is referred to in our popular culture as the balancing doctrine that the Supreme Court invokes in talking about the choice between individual freedom and the needs of the modern state.

I want to observe that Alexander Meiklejohn, in a marvelous little essay on the First Amendment, has pointed out that this balancing doctrine in our law has its origins in a profound error committed by Oliver Wendell Holmes. The Holmes notion of freedom of speech was predicated upon, as Meiklejohn said, "the vulgar notion of the marketplace"; he held that the First Amendment was addressed to the right of the citizen to be heard, to put his proposition into the "marketplace of ideas." Meiklejohn's correction of the Holmes error was to point out that the First Amendment was to protect the right of the individual to hear and to point out, further, that the citizen as the governor, as the sovereign of a self-governing democracy, must have absolute freedom with respect to the public business. It is this sanctity of the individual that is the end for which an open society exists. And so, I say, we cannot have any balancing of the integrity and sanctity of the individual against any need of society for increase in its knowledge and understanding. Walsh McDermott said most wisely yesterday that the rendering of informed consent, under whatever circumstances, cannot relieve the investigator of his solemn moral obligation and responsibility for the terms and conditions of his study.

JOAN GOLDSTEIN: I have been the National Coordinator of the Women's Health Task Force of the National Organization for Women. I speak as a feminist, as a sociologist, and hopefully, as a humanist.

One of the questions that has been raised this afternoon, and very well raised, is the one of role definition: that is, who are the persons who are used for human experimentation? We have the captive group, that is, the persons in institutions, mental institutions and prisons. We have the poor and, as Dr. Foster mentioned, also the Chicano women who were experimented on in terms of birth control. And so we would have to say "Women". Any woman who has been given an oral contraceptive has, in fact, been a subject in human experimentation.

Thus, the group seems to be a specific or special population group. It is not the large population; it is a special population on whom experimentation is done. We are led to believe that experimentation is done on persons for their benefit. Does that mean that they are the prized members of society because they would benefit more than anyone else from it?

I think the conclusion we would have to draw is that this is not the case. They are the expendable members of the society, not the privileged. My concern is not that there be federal regulations over the human experimentation, but that the federal regulations will not be enforced, that we will be led to believe that by virtue of this system we will be protected. Obviously, we need to be protected, because somehow or other we are the chosen people. So, therefore, I think my concern is that we focus a great deal more not only on regulatory recommendations, but that the enforcement and monitoring of such human experimentation, as well as data collection, which has been extremely poor in the whole area of birth control devices, be put into effect and mandated.

THOMAS: Thank you. I will take advantage of my position here at this podium simply to point out that there is a large population of patients on whom an intensive and, I would suggest, significant sort of clinical research is and has been going on for years in this country that has not been mentioned in comments either from the panels or the floor. These are people who are not imprisoned, not captive, and not in any way coerced, as far as I can see from my own experience. These are patients. Most of the work, for instance, that goes on these days on the problem of multiple sclerosis where clinical investigative questions arise is on using volunteer patients who have that particular disease. Most of the research effort now engaged countrywide in trying to find a more satisfactory answer to the problem of cancer is correspondingly being done on patients with cancer. I hate to make it seem as though that kind of research has come to an end, and that our main concern is how to do larger and larger scale research on normal human subjects.

D. T. CHALKLEY: I am from the National Institutes of Health, and I would like to give you a few statistics.

The NIH over the period since 1947 has supported about 80,000 research projects involving human subjects. Since it supports about one-third of the research, that means that there have been approximately one-quarter million projects involving human subjects supported in this country since roughly 1947.

In the last two days we have heard the litany -- Tuskegee, the Nazis, the Chicano women, Dr. Stough, and Dr. Mandel. Nobody has mentioned Sanger yet, nobody has mentioned Hodgman, and nobody has mentioned Dieckmann. Strangely, Willowbrook has been mentioned only briefly, but with no reference specifically to hepatitis and Shigellosis. Nobody has mentioned Holt's studies on infant nutrition, no reference to the cases in court at the moment -- Neilsen vs. Regents, Nelson vs. the United States, Baily vs. Mandel -- but they add up to about fifteen. That is .001 percent of all of the projects that have been supported in this country.

There were, in the last year, approximately 40,000 malpractice suits brought against the physicians in this country. Less than 2 percent of all physicians are engaged in research. Two percent of 40,000 would work out to about 800 expected malresearch cases; there are two in the courts. Nowhere in the entire history of American law has a malresearch suit been successfully prosecuted in a court in this country, not one. Yale University, a few years ago, looked into the question of whether or not their liability insurance could apply to malresearch as well as malpractice. Their insurance carrier looked into it and said, "Certainly," because there never had been a malresearch case. There have been instances, but they are rare.

One of the problems that we face in trying to equate all of this is the problem of the balancing provision that was referred to. There are, it is true, the First, the Fourth, and the Fifth Amendments, and surrounding these amendments the penumbra of informed consent. But against what do we balance this? Every national constitution set up in the twentieth century provides that the citizens have a right to medical care or access to medical care or even, in a couple of instances, a right to advances and improvements in medical care. Most of the constitutions set up in the nineteenth century have the same provision. But the Constitution of the United States was drawn in the eighteenth century, when it was believed that illness descended from on high through the Horsemen of the Apocalypse, and there was no mention of health anywhere in the United States Constitution.

Citizens of the Soviet Union have a right to medical care, but not the citizens of this country, not in the Constitution. Subjects of Elizabeth II, Queen of England, have a right to medical care and of access to medical care and improvements in medical care. But when in a constitutional situation one is required to balance the rights of consent, which are very real, against the individual, against the rights of the population to medical care, whether these persons be poor, whether they be prisoners or what have you, there is nothing against which one can constitutionally balance that question.

I would agree that an argument has been made very strongly over the past two days that research, if it is to be done, should be with and for the fetus, with and for children, with and for women, with and for the poor or any other group. What I see here is an argument over and over again that this group should be excluded, that group should be excluded, and I suspect that frankly all of us, sooner or later, would like to find reasons to exclude everybody. This is rapidly what we are getting to. But it is an old saying in the law that justice delayed is justice denied. It can equally truly be said in medicine that research delayed means benefits denied, and one of the problems we are facing is not only the balancing of the justice in the laws but the balancing of the medical rights of this community. I urge you to consider carefully the medical rights of those persons still here and still to become ill, and of those yet unborn, yet to be conceived who, if we do not consider research today, will suffer from those same diseases tomorrow.

ANDRE HELLEGERS: I am Director of the Joseph and Rose Kennedy Institute. Could I ask whether the health security imperative that is being postulated by Dr. Chalkley would be serious enough to institute a lottery type of draft to provide the population to be the subjects of the nontherapeutic research, and would that not then be a sort of general obligation of the public that would get us around all of the problems of special pleading for special works?

THOMAS: We will come back to that by way of the panel.

MARTIN KAPLAN: I am in charge of research development for the World Health Organization, Geneva, Switzerland. The particular point this morning is research on the poor. I merely wanted to urge that in formulating or improving and protecting the rights of the poor that the research involved not be displaced to foreign countries. One of the vulnerable population groups, as we all know, in many foreign developing countries are the poor. One particular area of research, the development of hyperimmune gamma globulin for antibody content by the plasma phoresis technique, has already found its place in certain of the poor countries where formerly it was done in the United States.

So, my plea would be that whatever safeguards are set up within the United States for the protection of its own poor also be taken into account for the poor of the other countries.

STEPHEN WELLS: I am a psychologist and a member of the Fordham-Yale Prison Research Project. I would like to address myself to the comments that Dr. Katz made concerning the interpersonal dynamics of the relationship that develops between researchers and subjects. I very much regretted not having the earlier opportunity to respond to Mr. Bronstein, who distorted our study and particularly with regard to the main thrust of the study, which was precisely on this point:

164

to examine the phenomenon of pharmacological research conducted in a prison from the standpoint of a psychological event and environment.

Our approach was to simulate a typical drug research experiment and then to evaluate it as one does a psychotherapeutic experience, to use standardized psychological measures both before and after. Our finding, which he neglected to mention because, I assume, it did not accord with his needs, was that we obtained highly significant changes in the direction of enhanced personal self-esteem and improved self-concept, with aggression diminished to a striking degree.

Granted, these were short-term findings and possibly not likely to endure. They did open the possibility that the very act of conducting research could be an experience that was highly beneficial for the subjects. This is the background on our present studies that have sought to examine this phenomenon in detail by constructing research environments modeled on therapeutic ones. We just finished a series of researches in the prison, and we are also going to be conducting these with free-living populations in which knowledge obtained from group therapy has been applied to the research setting. This would include educational experiences with regard to informing and informed consent, opportunities for extensive discussion on the part of subjects during the course of the experiment, as well as repeated opportunities to manifest consent, all of which has suggested to us that we are dealing with a much richer and more complex relationship than simply the act of an organism ingesting a substance for a certain purpose.

The possibilities of benefits, in terms of the experience that men have with accepting in positively oriented research the opportunity to generalize learning from an interest in the ongoing research, may be quite significant. Our conclusion from our research, among others, is that to have a mental health practitioner attached to a research unit to examine both the interaction between researchers and volunteers, and also to attempt to structure the environment so it is a beneficial one for the subjects, would be a useful addition to the present research practice. I would be interested if Dr. Katz would comment on that.

SABIN: This panel started out very well with definitions. Dr. Foster started out by saying that he wants a moratorium on medical research on the poor. He went on to define the poor as those who are illiterate, those who are senile, those who are mentally incompetent, or those who do not know English, and I suppose, do not have a translator at hand.

Now, I would like to make a comment about Dr. Katz. While Dr. Katz was talking, I was looking around the audience to see how many of my colleagues whom I know to be engaged or have been engaged in human medical research had horns sticking out of their forehead. I am quite sure that some scientists have horns, and so do others. I think philosophers commit mistakes, as well as lawyers, scientists,

and all other members of society, and we should be very careful
about those mistakes and to see that they do not occur.

Having said that, Dr. Katz posed a question from Isaiah Berlin:
Who in the name of what has the right to do anything to a person
without his consent? My answer to that very important question is
that the laws established by society and not by individuals have
that right; but as Abraham Lincoln long ago said, "There must be a
mechanism whereby laws that are bad can be repealed or modified."
We can specify for future guidance the definition that Dr. Foster
gave, and we should not generalize from the few mistakes to all.
The colleagues that I know are as much members of that large group
who respect human rights and the rights of the individuals as that
small group who have erroneously appropriated to themselves that
name which belongs to the hundreds of millions of decent people in
the world.

BERNARD BARBER: I am a sociologist and have done some research in this
field. I would like to address myself to Dr. Chalkley and especially, also, to those who applauded so vigorously at his remark.
First of all, as to the facts, he is alleging that only fifteen out
of 250,000 projects supported by the NIH since 1947 have been -- I
was going to say actionable at law -- have been taken to the courts.
The data from our study actually showed that something like about 10
percent, by the evidence of the researchers' own responses and the
researchers' own definitions, have not conformed to proper standards
of informed consent or risk-benefit ratio. First of all, the facts
are such that there is a greater problem here than Dr. Chalkley is
saying.

But I am more distressed by the stance that he is taking and that
the medical researchers are taking. Do you mean to tell me, do you
mean to tell yourself that your definition is now going to be legality rather than morality? Do you mean to tell me that the medical
research profession in this country, which for the last thirty or forty
years claimed to be in a somewhat higher moral position than the
therapeutic medical profession, is not about to place itself in the
same position as the medical therapeutic group? Do you want 40,000
malresearch suits? If you don't, if you are going to stand on
morality, we have to start doing something about it now. Nobody is
accusing you of having horns.

People are saying that there is a new moral climate. We need
your help. We have to work together. We have to do something about
all of this. A simple negative defensiveness will not do. I insist
that one of the great reservoirs of morality in this country has
been the biomedical research profession, and I very much hope that
in this new moral task that confronts us that strength will not be
given up.

JAMES CHILDRESS: I am Chairman of the Department of Religious Studies
at the University of Virginia. Following Mr. Piel, I, too, want to

166

call into question the doctrine of balancing individual risk and
societal benefits, not so much in a legal sense as in a social and
moral sense. I want to suggest that there is a more fundamental
question in back of it, one that actually determines how we proceed.
What are our starting points? What are our presumptions or, to use
legal-like language, who has the burden of going forward and who
has the burden of proof, and what is the burden of proof?

Now, I would suggest that there are two models that work in our
discussion. One model that we have heard, perhaps most frequently
from the researchers, gives as a starting point the great benefits
of medical research. The presumption is that it will achieve benefits. Then one asks how and within what limits, perhaps with a
certain fear of restrictions, especially governmental restrictions.

A second model, and one that I would propose, starts with a
different presumption. It is that we should not engage in nontherapeutic experimentation on human beings and do not impose risk on
subjects if those risks cannot bear benefit and unless certain information cannot be gained in any other way. I would use the language of necessity, and would also add "unless there can be consent."
Then I would want to see the procedures to enforce this.

In actual practice there will certainly be agreement between
these two models relating to many cases, perhaps even to most cases.
But I think what one sees as important issues will depend to a great
extent on the starting points and presumptions, and to talk about
balancing apart from them is to misunderstand the issue.

VIJAYA MELNICK: I am a faculty member in the Department of Biology at
the Federal City College. First of all, I would like to make the
comment that since I see Dr. Foster on the platform, I am finally
happy to see some color on this podium. Secondly, I read in the
program that this is an Academy Forum on "Experiments and Research
with Humans: Values in Conflict." During the time that I have been
here conflict has been kept out; at least by the people who have
presented their papers from the platform, there is minimal conflict.
Yesterday there was hardly any. I question why the people who have
publicly held opposing views on these subjects, such as consumer
groups, student medical groups and so forth, those who have been
involved in poverty research, as well as in concerns in the poverty
area, have not been invited or been part of this presentation. I
think that we have to get more of a total point of view, and if we
were really interested in finding out the various points of view
that we should have had those represented on this platform.

LOUIS LASAGNA: I am Professor and Chairman of the Department of Pharmacology, University of Rochester School of Medicine and Dentistry. I
have long been persuaded that it is possible to do bad research and
stupid research and improper research on the rich and the poor and
blacks and whites and men and women and prisoners and nonprisoners.
I am also, however, persuaded that it is possible to do proper and

intelligent and socially useful research on almost any population that has been discussed during this two-day Forum. It seems to me what we should be doing is evolving rules for playing this game in such a way that things are done properly and ethically and with humanity and compassion.

I am struck by the fact that the horrors that are described, the giving of placebos to Chicano women or the injections of cancer cells into unknowing, chronically ill patients in Brooklyn or the horrors described at Nuremberg, perhaps have an added special dimension of horror by reason of the fact that the experiments involved the poor or Chicanos or Jews or prisoners. But I submit to you that these experiments are horrors independent of the nature of the population group. I submit to you that they would have been ethically improper and horrible were they done on Dr. Hubbard's family or the Rockefellers. Therefore, I think it behooves us to pay more attention to evolving rules that will be applicable to all, to the rich, the poor, the white and the black, the advantaged and the disadvantaged.

BERNARD DAVIS: I think Mr. Barber brought up a very important point in suggesting that the medical profession should not be happy at defending its actions simply in terms of the small number of legal attacks on research activities. I think this is a very fundamental point, because the whole movement that led to this Forum arose not many years ago when the field of medical ethics, which has always been implicit in medical practice since time immemorial, was taken out of the hands of doctors by professional ethicists and people with other backgrounds related to this who raised very serious questions of ethics, who helped sharpen the perception of doctors to errors that have crept into many research studies. For the first couple of years, as long as the discussions were concerned with sharpening the moral perceptions, this caused groups to be more self-conscious in medical research about the rights and wrongs of what we are doing. I think there would be few medical researchers that would not welcome that movement.

Now, however, what started as a concern with moral issues has become an increasing concern with legal actions. The promulgation of regulations that bind the medical profession, whether within the NIH or elsewhere, are legal actions. Dr. Edelin, for the last few weeks or months, has not been wrestling with a moral problem; he has been wrestling with a legal problem. I think that what leads to the polarization that I deplored in my remarks yesterday is that we are facing not only adversary relations in our discussions between certain lawyers and doctors; we are facing actions that are soon going to lead to extensive bureaucratization in the form of legislation. The dangers of legislation displacing moral concerns are those that all of us who wish to benefit from medicine must be worried about.

THOMAS: I would like to commend the panel for being so courageous and patient during all this time and now turn the meeting back to you.

FOSTER: My problem is compounded, as you can see. Not only do I have
to be concerned about whatever rules, regulations, guidelines are
structured for the whole realm of human experimentation, but I have
to be a bit more concerned as they are applied to both the poor and
to the blacks. I think everyone here realizes there is an asymmetri-
cal application of standards in this country. The likelihood of the
Hubbard family being ripped off is much less than for a poor black
family in this country. I am very sensitive to the fact that the
great majority of heart recipients have been white, and the donors
have been black. I know, and I feel it. For these reasons I am
trying to structure at least a segment or glean out from that population and protect those that are at most risk or most vulnerable.
I think this is appropriate; but again I would like to emphasize
that I think it is in the best interests of both science and the
humane community.

   I am in agreement with you, Dr. Katz, that the poor are quite
capable of comprehension. But many times they don't comprehend, not
from inherent deficiencies, but from deficiencies of the experimenters, rather than the experimentees. Things are not explained to
them, and no effort is made to do so. And indeed, there is an element of subterfuge often used because people may reject experimental
processes. But I really recommend my changes on different grounds.
I am concerned, as I have just mentioned, about the mal-application
of the standards and the lack of enforcement, and that is really
what prompts my recommendations.

KATZ: I want to be brief, and I don't know where to begin. I have a
hopeless feeling that we have not understood each other. If what I
talked about can be summed up in making the point that researchers
have horns, then I almost want to leave on the next plane.

   Researchers don't have horns. It would be nice if some of them
did because then we could identify them, and we would have no problem. But we are dealing here with really fundamental human, psychological, scientific, and value issues, difficult issues. I don't
think they can be resolved easily. And when I suggested that we
take one approach, I only did this in order to create some discussion. But I was more interested in saying that these value conflicts have to be acknowledged, and they were not acknowledged by
this Forum in this last day and one-half. For better or for worse
the research community feels under attack, and it had to take a
completely defensive attitude today and yesterday rather than to
explore the issue.

   I have two more very brief points. One is the horrors of the
experiments. I wish I had not even alluded to some of the horrible
experiments that I did. Dr. Lasagna is quite right: these horrible
experiments will occur under whatever regulations you might have.
The real problem is the day-to-day conduct of human research, and
what I wanted to open up for discussion is the extent to which human
subjects are not being informed that they are participating in a

research project. I can give you countless examples of their being lied to about the nature of the research, et cetera.

And this brings me to my final point, and I feel badly that it has to be ad hominem, but I do have to indemnify Dr. Chalkley. Dr. Chalkley, of course, is quite correct. Out of all these experiments only fifteen or so went to court in the last ten years; but if he does not know to what extent even the research projects that are being conducted under HEW guidelines are in violation of these guidelines, he ought to find out.

Of course, he cannot find out very easily or could not until recently. I am not sure whether the regulations have been changed. They change so fast these days that even I cannot keep up with them. But at least until recently there were not mechanisms in the HEW regulations that made it mandatory, for example, to report to him and to report to the Secretary whatever violations occurred in the conduct of research. But I think there is lots of it going on. Maybe it has to go on. I am not at all suggesting that things ought to be changed, not necessarily so. But we ought to be a little bit more self-conscious, and we ought to know a little bit more as to what we are doing and why we are doing it.

INGELFINGER: I agree with Dr. Barber that the medical research profession should not engage in negative defensiveness. But having said that, let me engage in a little bit of it, because you know you face facts. Dr. Thomas, yesterday, said, "I don't believe that all this outrageous experimentation goes on." Jay Katz now has said that he knows of many, many examples where patients are being lied to, where they are not being told about the nature of the experiment.

The editor of a medical journal cannot tell whether or not the subjects were lied to. So, I am not commenting on that. In the *New England Journal of Medicine*, if we now receive a paper of a randomized trial, we ask the author, "Did you or did you not tell the patients that the medication or the procedure you get is received by lot or was determined by lot?" So things are improving, I think, as a result of the efforts of many of the people who are here and others. This is a position we have taken, and people will be informed better.

To go back to negative defensiveness. Of course we should have a positive approach, but what is it? How can we achieve it? Can we achieve it by lottery? I think Dr. Hellegers was probably speaking with tongue in cheek; but no, I think one has to sell to the public. That is why I tried to make the point about more and more people being involved as administratively eligible subjects. One has to sell to the public the idea that medical research is ultimately beneficial. If people say that it isn't, then one cannot talk to them. But if it is, then one has to sell to the feminist, for example, the idea that she wants studies on contraceptives.

And Dr. Foster, if you want to exclude certain groups, the poor, all right; but you are going to deprive those poor of studies that are particularly germane to their problems. They are susceptible because of their economic deprivation to conditions of malnutrition or certain infections or other conditions, such as psychiatric problems. So, I think to exclude them from that kind of study is disadvantageous to them. I would hope that the poor would eventually push for certain studies. So, the positive approach that should come out of a meeting like this, I hope, would be a greater acceptance of the public for the need for medical research but under certain controlled conditions, which I agree should be a matter of ten commandments rather than a series of infinite numbers of small rules.

I should like to conclude by referring to an article by Hans Jonas in the 1969 issue of *Daedalus*, which I think is one of the best articles ever written in this general area and in which he covers practically all the subjects we have discussed in the last two days and in which, even though he is a philosopher, he does bring in the fact of balances. Dr. Jonas cites the following as the principle of the order of preference: "The poorer in knowledge, motivation, and freedom of decision, (and that, alas, means the more readily available in terms of numbers and possible manipulation), the more sparingly and indeed reluctantly should the reservoir be used, and the more compelling must therefore become the countervailing justification."

This, it seems to me, is the proper approach, namely, we don't make absolute rules. We do not prohibit use of captive groups, poor groups; but the more we use them, the more we have to know what we are doing, and the more careful we have to be in the implementation of our investigation.

REGULATORY, JUDICIAL, AND LEGISLATIVE PROCESSES

REMARKS BY THE HONORABLE
CASPAR W. WEINBERGER

Secretary of Health, Education,
and Welfare

The interest of the Department of Health, Education, and Welfare in the
issues that you are considering in this Forum is self-evident. A major
goal of the Department is to improve health through research; and
another is to protect the rights of those who participate in that research as subjects.

Some feel that this is an irreconcilable conflict. To us it represents only the necessity for achieving a reasonable balance of all of
the interests. In searching out this balance, we cannot forget that
no matter what various perspectives we bring to this task, there is
one common interest that we all share: the absolute necessity of continuing all forms of research and in such a way that the basic human
rights of all concerned are protected. If we forget either part of
that equation there will be very serious difficulty for us all, and for
mankind in general.

It would be foolish to suppose that there are no problems in doing
this or that it can be done easily. But it would be equally foolish to
suppose that we should not make the effort or that there can be no
progress, for we have actually already demonstrated rather substantial
progress. Fifteen years ago, HEW funded a study on clinical research
involving human subjects. That study, conducted by the Law and Medicine Institute at Boston University, cited a certain research project
in which investigators did spinal taps on healthy newborn infants without the parents' consent. The physicians who conducted this experiment saw nothing wrong with it at that time. They believed that as
physicians they were the best judges of whether the spinal taps were
safe or not. They said that parents could not possibly understand the
nature of their research, and therefore would probably deny their consent if asked. Such reasoning would be unthinkable now.

The issue today has advanced to new grounds. It now hinges on the
issue of whether informed consent from parents for a procedure that may
be of no immediate medical benefit to the infant, or perhaps ever, is
ethically acceptable and legally valid. The future of a great deal of
vital drug research also hinges on the resolution of this question.
These are things that necessarily have to be decided by a wide spectrum
in the community. I think that the best way to do it is to try to get
some as effective and as flexible guidelines as possible so that each
individual question does not have to be researched and tried out, so to
speak, and worked over at endless length while we are denied the fruits
of what could be and in many cases will be very valuable, very essential research.

On drugs there is a particular dilemma that I face and that will
illustrate some of the problems involved. The Harrison-Kefauver Act
declares that no drug to be used in interstate commerce can be advertised for use by any age group without first having identified the
correct dosage and both the safety and the efficacy of that drug. The
drugs now can be tested among adult volunteers, of course, to ascertain
those things. But if there is no way of trying to test drugs on children to get that kind of information -- and at the moment the mechanisms are, at least, cloudy -- new drugs could be denied to children
simply because there is no mechanism for prior testing. So, there is
no real way to abide by the Harrison-Kefauver Act as it applies to
drugs for children unless we get a clear mandate on the ethical issue
of testing drugs on children as subjects. As Secretary of the Department, I am obviously on the horns of the dilemma. I am responsible for
promulgating food and drug laws effectively, carrying them out, and
administering them, and yet we must certify that the Food and Drug
Administration is complying with the law. This would appear to be prevented in the absence of certain clear ethical guidelines concerning
the issues of how you get informed consent, how you can make some tests
on children and infants who, necessarily, have to be involved if we are
to develop the proper dosage, if we are to enable children to have the
benefits of what might be a very considerable medical advance. So, we
do need, obviously, to try to work out some kind of guidelines, some
kind of formulae that will enable us to conclude that there has been
sufficient informed consent to proceed.

There is no body of law -- statutory or case law or constitutional
law -- that clarifies or gives us a certain answer on this whole problem of informed consent. So the needs of science and the needs of
humanity have moved, in a sense, beyond the present insights of the
law. But since, as Mr. Justice Holmes said, "The life of law is
experience," we may very well hope that the experiences can become part
of the law. That is essentially the process in which we are engaged
right at this precise moment.

Who can give informed consent for minors in research projects? The
law likes to reason from analogies, and we have some analogies in
guardianship cases, matters that are not quite as important as this in
many situations, but some that might be considered. There are those

where we recognize that infants and in some cases unborn children cannot give that consent, where we recognize that consent of children is necessary and we try to find somebody who can at least be a sufficiently close representative with sufficiently close interests so that they will be able to substitute for the child until he achieves maturity and the ability to give an informed consent. That is a familiar enough thing in the law in other situations. We can perhaps use some of those analogies to develop further guidelines.

Drugs, of course, are not the only problem here. Also at issue is the whole progress of research, for example, into the chronic degenerative diseases. As scientists, you will know far more than I about the fact that the most vital area of research against heart disease and cancer is concerned with investigations of normal tissues, normal bodies, all of the development that might be considered normal, in order to define abnormal. For this purpose, obviously, research must be conducted among a population of presumably normal infants, normal adults, normal volunteers. In order to conduct that research, we have to find some means of developing a method that protects the interests of those infants and children whom we are investigating to see if, in fact, they are normal. This, in turn, can help us produce happier, healthier lives for millions of individuals not yet born who also have an interest that has to be represented; and in many cases is represented to some extent, by the people doing the research. So it is a classic kind of dilemma involved in public administration and ethics and law and science. There is no question that this kind of work has to be done.

Another very hot, burning issue in this whole field is the use of prisoners for research. Scientists have long viewed prisoners as an ideal population for certain controlled studies, because their diets and their life-styles are easily observed and easily controlled. As you know, many very beneficial discoveries, particularly in the fields of immunization and microbiological processes, have come from research on prisoner subjects. I think it is clear that they are needed in many kinds of research. What is not clear is whether or how prisoners, who live in a coercive environment, can freely give their informed consent to become research subjects. This is an issue about which there is little likelihood of any final agreement, and the matter certainly has not been helped by some of the more recent examples that have been before us and that started many, many years ago. I don't know that we are ever going to get a solution in which we can say that everyone believes there has been full and final agreement or that is the proper way to protect the interests of prisoners. Some would say that the only way you could do that is to make sure that they are released from prison, at which point you lose all of the biological advantages of having them in a controlled environment. But we must come to some kind of reasonable decision on the question. I don't think it is reasonable to say that the situation is too difficult or too delicate and therefore that we should not consider it, because there are very real and very necessary advantages to this kind of population. But it is equally important that we make every effort to get what in many cases is a somewhat easier way than is the case with infants and children, a truly informed consent; and the voluntary nature of it, of course, is the place in which a lot of this would start.

This illustrates, I think, the reason why, at one time, it seemed to me so obvious that it was going to be virtually impossible, in this or in some of the other governmental tasks that I have tried to perform, to please everyone. Now I am being brought rapidly to the conclusion that it is going to be impossible to please anyone. Nevertheless, that would certainly not be a deterrent for trying because the stakes are too high. The goals are too necessary, and the results are too hopeful to allow us to give up.

So solutions are a very real necessity. The real test will be whether the compromises that inevitably will have to be made to bring us to a final result will safeguard the essential rights and responsibilities of everyone concerned, and yet ensure that researchers will have sufficient freedom to continue making at least attempts to secure and duplicate the illustrious achievements of the past.

It is easy enough to state the dilemma. But this is essential, because if we don't, it is too easy to say that one factor overrides everything else, and therefore we can ignore everything else. If we don't state that dilemma, if we don't realize the difficulty of the problem, then I think we tend to polarize and to prevent and in effect make much more difficult our ultimate task.

We have made a substantial amount of progress, I think. In 1966, the then Surgeon General issued a policy statement governing the protection of human subjects in projects that were supported by the Public Health Service. The policy was codified in what you call and know as "The Yellow Book." I am told that when that first was published, some scientists said that the code would simply make impossible any future research because of red tape and delays. This is not to say that the Yellow Book was perfect or that the guidelines can now be picked up and followed in all programs, but those dire predictions did not come true. In many ways, the 1960s turned out to be a golden decade for scientific inquiry, and I think that a great deal of it was done accompanied by and guarded by some of the protections that were first proposed in the mid-sixties. Once you bring the ghosts out of the closet and look at some of the problems and some of the difficulties, approaching them on a kind of one-by-one basis or step-by-step basis, to quote from a colleague of mine in the Cabinet, it is quite possible to get solutions that initially seem to be impossible.

We should not underestimate the difficulties. They are very real. But sometimes I think that we make some of our own difficulties just by believing that they are too hard to overcome. A few years ago the Director of the National Institutes of Health began several studies to develop guidelines for protecting prisoners and the mentally retarded when they were involved in NIH-supported research. In time the scope of these studies embraced all activities that were conducted by the Department. Eventually, a few months ago, this resulted in my issuing proposed policy and draft regulations to govern research involving these special subjects. Misunderstanding and suspicion have arisen over some of these proposals. I think this is not a bad time to try to clear up some of these.

The first point, I think, that should be made is that we did not issue these proposals in reaction to congressional prodding. Our work preceded by a long time the interest of the Congress. I don't think that is particularly important, but I mention it only because a lot of people have said, "Well, you did not really mean this. You just rushed into it because the Congress forced you to do so." Some people say that we never do anything that the Congress wants us to do anyway. So this would be sort of inconsistent with that viewpoint. But the simple fact is that the Department, for a long time before I came and while I have been there, has been very interested and deeply concerned with the necessity of trying to deal with this problem of protection while permitting and encouraging necessary research.

Secondly, these proposals did not emerge from the perspectives of some narrow interest group. This, again, is a curious example of the way the attacks normally come. Some said that they were the work of prople who had no training in research and who had a built-in bias against having any done. Others said quite the opposite, that all of these things came from apologists for the research community, and therefore were automatically to be distrusted. The facts are -- and I know because I participated in a great many of the sessions, having a real interest in this subject myself -- that the people who put these proposals together represented a balance of interests and expertise. There were lawyers, including myself and many others. There were research scientists, and we had a person trained in bioethics, which is a comparatively new field, but one which we thought was very important to have represented. These people, in turn, consulted at length with some of the nation's most respected experts in law, medicine, and ethics, many of whom, I am happy to note, are present today. There was a sustained effort made to try to get many differing viewpoints and many of the interests that have to be balanced brought into consideration during the course of this process.

The real problem is not any lack of sensitivity to competing interests, but it is this very difficult task of trying to balance and reconcile diverse and strongly held views on both sides, stating the terms of that reconciliation in ways that will permit us to administer future regulatory programs fairly without looking at each single research experiment and applying some kind of different, perhaps subjective, standard to it.

There is another example that might be of interest. One of our proposed regulations would require any research conducted overseas with our government funds to comply with the essential standards of the policy as a whole. That, I think, is a broad way to phrase it, but it is a clear indication of what is desired and what is intended. However, it also provides, as I think you have to do, that under special circumstances the policies can be modified. We have had a lot of differences over this proposal. Some say that it is wrong for our government to

attempt to dictate to other nations how our research should be conducted in their countries. Others say that any opportunity or any possibility of modifying the requirements would merely drive unethical
research overseas. The real problem, however, is to assure that all of
our funded research meets with our basic ethical standards, while admitting that some conditions make strict adherence to all parts of the
regulations frankly impossible.

We have one case, just as an example, although there are obviously
going to be many others. If a research project were planned to dis-
tribute a nutritional supplement to a group of tribes in an African
country, would it be reasonable for that investigator to be required to
convene a consent committee composed of a lawyer, a physician, a community representative, and an ethicist to determine whether it should
be done? I think just stating that indicates the impossibility of it.
But under the model that we have talked about we think it would be
possible to consider such cases on their merits, and that is the value
of the review procedures that we propose. We could not achieve the
necessary degree of flexibility if the program were established by
congressional act or a court order, which is quite likely. And court
orders are much more likely to be rather totally negative than to have
any degree of flexibility.

So, what we are trying to do is to develop some kind of a set of
safeguards that will have a broader application than just a single
individual project, that will have some degree of flexibility, that will
enable this vital research to continue, and that will enable us to be
able to assure the public -- as indeed we have to do -- that human
rights are indeed being protected. I don't think we can ignore this
point at all because the public, through Congress and through numerous
other bodies, has voiced its interest and its concern. Since that is
the kind of government we have, fortunately, it is clear that the
establishment of any kind of public rules for the conduct of research
involving human subjects is public business. For one thing, it is
funded with public funds to a very considerable extent, and it is something that is obviously going to have to have the support of the public.
It is the province of no one group that is narrower or smaller than the
public as a whole. The issues are the province of no one. They are
the concern of everyone -- the scientist, the research subject, the
taxpayer, and the public who are ultimately to be the beneficiaries of
the findings of that scientific research.

Another way of saying it is that if you are to have publicly supported research, it does, indeed, have to be publicly supported. You
do have to have considerations of this kind clearly in mind, and I
think everyone has to recognize their vital importance. So I particularly welcome, and I am sure everyone here as well as everyone in the
scientific community who may not be here will welcome, the creation of
the National Commission for the Protection of Human Subjects of Biomedical and Behavioral Research that we chartered and held opening
meetings for just a few weeks ago.

This Commission has agreed to undertake a very difficult and perhaps a thankless job. But we chose as carefully as we could to try to get not only a high degree of expertise but a broad representation of the interests that do, indeed, have to be balanced. I think without the public spirited work of this Commission, the work of everyone in science might well come to a standstill. That would be bad for everyone, and most especially the prople who are destined to benefit from research.

We should be clear on one thing: the work of this Commission is your work, everyone's work. Its success is either going to be your success or your failure. The health and well-being of countless millions, including many unborn generations whose interests cannot be represented on that side any more than they can be directly represented on the side of whether they can consent, will depend on the work of this Commission. I hope it will have your support, your understanding, and your cooperation.

I would like to express the deep appreciation that I feel to the National Academy of Sciences for its initiative in convening this Forum. Your deliberations will help to provide an invaluable and essential backdrop for those of the Commission. They will enormously help me and all of may colleagues in the Department. I would be astounded if there is full agreement, but I would be equally disappointed if there are not some extraordinarily valuable contributions made that will benefit the National Commission, but more importantly, perhaps, in the longer range will benefit all of mankind.

INQUIRY AND COMMENTARY

PHILIP HANDLER: Thank you very much, Mr. Secretary, for this very thoughtful and illuminating statement. We are most grateful. Secretary Weinberger has indicated his willingness to answer a few questions.

SECRETARY WEINBERGER: I hope they will all be of a suitable technical difficulty so that I will be able to display my layman's qualities.

GEORGE HILL: I am not sure I will be technical or suitable, but I will try. Mr. Weinberger, why is it that you pick on the poor and the poverty people to get the brunt of the cutoffs in Medicaid and the various programs that have come through many years of hard labor and decisive fighting of our congressmen for them? Why do you insist on destroying the benefits of the poor and those who are too weak to assert their prerogatives in Congress? Is there, perhaps, some feeling on your part that they are not the deserving poor?

180

WEINBERGER: That question is so totally incorrect in its assumptions
that while it is obviously, I am sure, an important part of your
agenda this afternoon, I will nevertheless answer. We have a $1.6
billion increase in Medicare and Medicaid, and even in these times,
and even by Washington standards, I would not consider that that is
cutting off or destroying a program.

HILL: I don't think you have answered my question. At the prices that
we in Medicaid have to pay there is a great discrepancy between what
you speak of in total numbers of dollars and what each poor individual has to spend for medicine.

WEINBERGER: That is not correct. At a $1.6 billion increase, we are
well ahead of even today's much too high rate of inflation, and
there will be real benefit increases in both programs.

HILL: No physician wants to take a Medicaid applicant or dependent.
How will you arrange to develop a program in which more money --

HANDLER: I am sorry, sir, but you have departed from the subject of the
meeting.

WEINBERGER: Fortunately, several physicians are more than willing and
eager and happy to take Medicare and Medicaid patients.

DENIS PRAGER: I am Director of the Population Studies Center at
Battelle Memorial Institute. Mr. Secretary, one of the problems
that many of us face is the protection of the institutions doing
medical research. On the one hand, we are attempting to use our
institutional committees to protect the rights and welfare of human
subjects. On the other hand, if many of the institutions do not
obtain some sort of an indemnification, we will be unable to take
the kinds of risks institutionally that are necessary. My understanding is that at least in your Department, it is the prerogative
of the Secretary himself to grant these kinds of indemnification. I
wonder what kinds of things are happening within the Department?

WEINBERGER: That is a very good question, and it touches a very difficult point. If we can work out the set of guidelines and rules
under which it would be clear that research conducted according to
certain well-understood guidelines did not produce liability, we
would not reach the question of indemnification because you would
not have to indemnify anyone except against a liability.
    Now, this is not to say that there might be people working under
the auspices of an institution who might depart from those guidelines. Then you would have your normal agency rules and all the
rest as to whether or not the institution was ultimately liable.

What I would like to try to do would be to work out indemnification primarily where there has been a following of the guidelines that are laid out. In other words, I would like the guidelines to be so clear, both to the institution and to the person doing the research, that the ways of doing it are stated and can easily be followed. If there is a departure from that and the institution is in no way responsible, then without any action by the Secretary and in the normal course the institution would possibly be freed from liability by the courts.

The difficulty is, as we know, that anybody can be sued for anything regardless of the merits of the case. And the expense of defending is very great. If I had not spent most of this morning dealing with what we, I think, correctly call the malpractice crisis, I would suggest that possibly one of the better ways to try to do it would be through some form of insurance. After this morning's session, I am not entirely sure that that is correct. But we would try our best to insure that both the institution where the work is done -- because obviously they have to be encouraged to do it and to sponsor it -- and the individual who does it, if they follow certain guidelines, would be freed of later responsibility. That indeed would be the purpose of the guidelines. And this argues for trying to make the guidelines as clear, as easily understandable, and as easy to follow as we can. It adds to the size of the problem, but I do not think in any sense that it is insoluble. It is handled in analogous ways in other legal situations throughout the whole spectrum of the economy.

SAMUEL GOROVITZ: I am Chairman of the Department of Philosophy, University of Maryland. I think it can be argued that although universities have no monopoly on good quality research, the possibility of maintaining productive research programs of the sort that we all desire depends very importantly on the maintenance of vigorous, viable, and diverse universities. Yet higher education in this country today is in a very tenuous condition. Its financial base is rapidly eroding. Many institutions are on the brink of collapse. There does not seem to be in the near future any obvious solution. I wonder if you would comment on the views of your office and the plans to resolve this difficulty.

WEINBERGER: Well, obviously any organization that spends in excess of $5.5 billion on the subject is interested in it. And it is clearly, as you say, an extraordinarily important part of the entire subject. We are very interested in it. We are aware of the difficulties and the ravages of inflation on higher education and on some of the problems that are involved in suitable student assistance and in institutional aid. We do think that, first of all, we have very substantial student assistance programs before the Congress. We

believe that that is one of the very best ways of ensuring the continuum of expertise and skills and continued existence of many of
the universities and institutions of higher education. Student
assistance we think is a very proper way to go and a preferable
way to proceed, rather than simply trying to divide the resources
that are available -- and they are limited, as all resources are --
among all institutions in some kind of a roughly equal formula. So
we have opted for increased student assistance, both at the under-
graduate as well as at the graduate level.

We obviously will continue to fund a number of research projects
of a substantial nature. The obvious place for carrying out these
research projects will be institutions that are equippped to do so
and have the skilled personnel, many of whom will have been trained
with federal government assistance to carry them out. So this will
be another source of federal funding.

In the final analysis, we will continue to rely on very substantial state support for public higher educational institutions, as
we have had in the past. Here again I should emphasize the point
that I mentioned earlier: these publicly supported institutions
have to have public support. So there will be considerations of
matters in which the public is extremely interested, as the ones you
were considering. This is not to say that we are going to tell
them how to run themselves. That would be the very last thing that
I would want to do. It is a thing that I think the government is
singularly ill-equipped to do, aside from any moral or philosophical
factors involved. But there will have to be considerations by the
institutions themselves of the need for maintaining public support
if they are to encourage the kinds of public contributions from
state and local funds that have been there in the past and I am sure
will be there in the future.

Ultimately we are going to have to reduce very sharply the totally
unacceptable rate of inflation that is now in the economy and is
eroding not only the value of all that everyone does but, even worse,
is eroding public confidence in our institutions. The basic policy
of the government is designed to try to overcome that inflationary
spiral as quickly as we can. It is part of the dilemma. We can, as
a federal government, with $52 billion, $62 billion, and possibly
$70 billion deficits contribute mightily to more inflation. We
know that inflation hurts particularly the people our Department was
called into being to serve, hurts them more than any other group in
the community. It also hurts institutions and research projects.

These are all things that we have to have in mind as we try to
devise the basic policy of the government. I am convinced first of
all, that the importance of strong, healthy, growing universities
and postgraduate institutions is so vital for the future of the
country that it does now and always will occupy a very big part of
the priority setting of our Department and of any Administration.
But there are these other factors that I have mentioned that will
undoubtedly have to be considered in the course of it. But certainly

the placement of federal research, the training of research scientists, the institutional aid to some extent for specialties, heavy emphasis on student assistance at all levels -- these are keystones of our policy and certainly would be of the policy of most anyone who addressed these problems.

DORIS HAIRE: My interest is in maternal and child health. I find in dealing with the various Washington agencies that there seems to be a great reluctance in those agencies to alert women that virtually every woman in the United States who goes into the hospital to have a baby is an experimental animal. And there is almost no discussion about the fact that we know almost nothing about the long-term effects of these drugs. What agency can one go to to see that this information is given out to the general public?

WEINBERGER: It is the statutory task and the responsibility of the Food and Drug Administration to test with great care all new drugs; to continue to apply the latest technologies to old drugs that are authorized for general use; and to report to physicians, hospitals, the public, and all who would be concerned the effects of these drugs -- their good effects, what they might do, their possible negative effects, and so on. In order to be able to carry out those responsibilities, some experimentation, as I have indicated, is clearly required.

I personally think it is overstating it a bit to say that everyone who enters the hospital to have a baby is a human experiment. There are so many procedures that are so thoroughly accepted and understood and followed so regularly that they can be said to have passed beyond the experimental stage. If there are new drugs or drugs that are not formally and officially approved by the Food and Drug Administration and that are proposed to be used, then clearly there should be the fullest and most complete understanding of that by the patient, by the doctor, by the hospital, followed by agreement or refusal to permit their use.

We obviously are trying to improve. But we do and should rely and have to rely on the assignment that the Congress has made to the Food and Drug Administration to carry out its responsibilities in this field. The use that is made of the information that is available on the label and in the various publications obviously cannot be controlled directly by the government, nor should it be. But the information is there. It is our duty to get it there, to get it accurately and completely and up to date, making use of all new things that we know and hear about and learn. Once that is done, if we are successful in our task of providing sufficient protections in the use of any experiments of new drugs in order to acquire this basic data, then we will have proper consent for that.

That I think would be the best answer I could give. I would be surprised if there was general agreement that every woman who entered

184

a hospital to have a child was indeed a human research subject. But
I do think that it is necessary for situations where that is clearly
the case, where new drugs are being used, to have the protections
that we hope will come from the National Commission, from your
deliberations, from the careful concern and consideration of the
public over the next few months.

THE NATIONAL COMMISSION FOR THE PROTECTION OF HUMAN SUBJECTS OF BIOMEDICAL AND BEHAVIORAL RESEARCH

Charles U. Lowe

On July 12, 1974, the President signed an act now known as Public Law 93348, establishing a National Commission for the Protection of Human Subjects of Biomedical and Behavioral Research. I would like to discuss this piece of legislation with you and hopefully identify some special aspects of it that may not be immediately perceived by all of you.

This Commission, to which the Secretary alluded and which this Public Law creates, has, in my estimate, several major studies that it must undertake. First is a general discussion of the four principles that underlie our responsibilities in clinical research: the question of what is care and what is research; the assessment of what is risk and benefit when individuals are involved in clinical research; the necessity for identifying guidelines on how to select individuals for clinical research; and finally, perhaps the most difficult, the nature and definition of informed consent.

The second charge to the Commission deals with consideration of informed consent for a group of subjects who may indeed be unable to give informed consent for themselves. These are generally recognized to encompass the classes included when one says minors, prisoners, and the institutionalized mentally infirm. The Act does, however, add a fourth category which it could be argued are diminished in some way in their ability to give informed consent. These are those individuals who receive their care under programs conducted by or supported by the Secretary.

Another charge to the Commission, and a very difficult one, is to identify methods of protecting human subjects who are involved in biomedical or behavioral research that is in fact not funded and therefore not controlled by the Secretary of the Department of Health, Education, and Welfare.

The Commission also is charged to report to the Secretary and recommend policies defining the circumstances, if any, under which fetal research, research on the living fetus, may be conducted or supported.

Next, the Commission is charged to investigate and to study and to report to the Secretary the circumstances, if any, under which psychosurgery may be used.

And finally, the Commission is charged with the development of a very large study that attempts to identify technological advances, social response to these advances, ethical posture necessary to accommodate these advances, and public understanding of these advances. And within the scope of this large study, the Commission is to identify such public policy as must be advanced or identified to assist the public to accommodate to these changes. These constitute the visible charges to the National Commission.

I would now like to identify what I call the invisible charges, the hidden issues, or even the hidden agendas of the legislation.

First of all, that section of the Law that charges the Commission to identify the application of informed consent principles to individuals who are receiving health care services under programs conducted or supported by the Secretary sounds, on first reading, as if it concerns, for example, the Indians of the United States, whose total health care is provided by the Secretary. But if read carefully, it seems to me, it means that all individuals who are receiving health care within the United States are in effect covered by this particular paragraph since programs under the Hill-Burton Act, categorical health programs, Medicare, Medicaid, Professional Standards Review Organization, and Health Maintenance Organization are in fact all supported by the Department.

Another hidden agenda, as I call it, is in that section which charges the Commission to identify methods of protecting subjects who are involved in research not supported by the Department, and hence the Secretary has no direct authority over the programs. This indeed gets at the whole infrastructure of drug testing within the United States and particularly Phase III testing. It seems to me that it moves directly into the office of the physician who engages with a pharmaceutical manufacturer in a program or project to test a particular agent.

Finally, it is interesting that although the main thrust of the Commission is research, there is no mention of research with respect to psychosurgery. The issue is when should psychosurgery be used, when is it appropriate. In effect it charges the Commission with telling the Secretary how any behavior control achieved through psychosurgery should be administered, and in effect thus attempts to regulate a specific element of health care or medical practice. In general we have left these requirements to the individual states in their licensing procedures.

We now come to the special authorities contained in this legislation. In two instances the Commission is directed to report not to the

Secretary but directly to the Congress. These include that section in which the Commission is required to develop protection for subjects in research not funded by the Secretary, and the preparation of the agenda for the National Advisory Council for Protection of Subjects of Biomedical and Behavioral Research, which will be the surviving body after the two years of activity of the Commission have expired.

Another rather interesting authority contained within this Act is the fact that in contrast to other Congressional, Presidential, or Departmental Commissions, the Congress was unwilling to let the Commission deliberate and simply deliver its report. The Congress charged the Secretary with the Development of regulations to implement the recommendations of the Commission. Therefore, there is little chance that the report will simply sit on the shelf of some federal official or an interested public.

Finally, as the Congress apparently was concerned less the Commission act and then be dissolved, it established within this piece of legislation a National Council to advise the Secretary. This is to be a continuing body with no finite life to deal with all ethical issues as they emerge during progress in science and changes in biomedical technology.

I would now like to discuss the so-called fetal ban. In Section 213 of this Act, the Congress said, "Until the Commission has made its recommendations to the Secretary pursuant to Section 202(b)" -- which is the charge to evaluate fetal research per se -- "the Secretary may not conduct or support research in the United States or abroad on a living human fetus before or after the induced abortion of such fetus, unless such research is done for the purpose of assuring the survival of such fetus." I have quoted directly from the statute because it seems to me there is more misunderstanding about the so-called fetal ban than any other element in this particular piece of legislation.

The ban is quite specific. It is limited to living human fetuses, before or after induced abortion of such fetuses. And it is limited in time, four months; and it is limited in that it does not exclude any research done to ensure the survival of such fetuses. I might add parenthetically that it is not part of the legislation that the Department, in publishing its regulations relevant to this subsection of the Act, chose specifically to enforce only the language of the Act and has not created a total ban on fetal research. It is also worth noting that this particular section addresses only the authority of the Secretary of the Department of Health, Education, and Welfare. This is not a national or federal ban on fetal research. It relates only to such fetal research as specified in the Act and such fetal research as is supported by the Department of Health, Education, and Welfare.

I will conclude with two general observations. It is my judgment that this nation has in general, and perhaps even specifically, throughout its history, avoided all opportunities to sharpen controversial issues so that a head-to-head battle might ensue, in effect so that the strongest might totally subjugate the weaker. This is particularly true with respect to moral issues. The single exception that I can identify

188

was the question of slavery and its attendant evils and economic rami-
fications. The first half of the nineteenth century is replete with
political efforts to blunt the ethical questions surrounding slavery.
When these efforts finally failed and the opponents were apparently
exhausted by compromise, the issue crystallized and civil war ensued.
This is a lesson that cannot be lost on many who observe our present
efforts.

My second observation is that traditionally we have, I believe, in
this country avoided legislating moral issues, and even from time to
time, particularly with respect to the original states, removed from
the statute books laws that smacked of sectarian interest: for example,
the repeal of Blue Laws. We are now, for better or for worse, committed
to a process that in fact may eventuate in regulating ethics. The
approach is indirect in that the apparatus is administrative and regulatory rather than legislative and judicial. But in my judgment we are
set in this course and in fact have initiated a major national experiment. How well and how successfully our Commission moves to confront
this challenge remains to be seen. But the tranquility of the nation
and the emotional temperature may well be affected by its deliberations.

REGULATORY, JUDICIAL, AND
LEGISLATIVE PROCESSES

The Panel:

Charles Fried
Maurice R. Hilleman
Richard A. Merrill

CHARLES FRIED

In the segment of this program which is devoted in part to a consideration of legal regulation of fetal research I must take thirty seconds
from my prepared remarks to say this. Whatever one's moral convictions
regarding abortion, I think we should all condemn the prosecution and
conviction of a doctor who, in good faith, performed an abortion to
which the United States Supreme Court has said that the pregnant woman
involved was constitutionally entitled. This prosecution and conviction are an obvious perversion of justice and a lawless act. It brings
shame and disgrace on all of those associated with it. No one of us,
no matter what his convictions or sect, is safe if the criminal law can
be twisted in this shameful and cynical way.

In the last decade there has been an immense growth of interest,
writing, regulatory material, and bureaucratic time devoted to regulation of experimentation with human subjects. It is striking that the
NIH guidelines and the recent regulations have by and large not proposed any new principles to govern this topic except in certain special
cases, such as fetal research, to which I shall come presently.

I do not mean to suggest that the principles in those guidelines and
regulations are not splendid, only that they do not in any sense inno-
vate. The basic concepts can be found in the ancient principles of the
law. The concept of battery has traditionally protected the integrity
of the person from interferences with his body and has permitted such
interferences only when there is consent. That concept of consent has
traditionally meant freely given consent, informed consent, untainted
by fraud or concealment. Similarly, the law of negligence has always
required an inquiry into the proper ratio of risks and benefits in

189

determining whether conduct leading to injury was reasonable. Both of these families of concepts have been widely applied to the area of medical treatment, although the number of cases involving medical research have been very few indeed. Dr. Chalkley has told us this morning that they are none. In a little byplay between us I think he has almost persuaded me.

Finally there is another concept of wide and traditional application that should cover the experimental situation. And that is the notion of the fiduciary relationship. A lawyer, an accountant, a trustee, a guardian, a corporate officer or a corporate director are all fiduciaries for those whose interests they can affect and who rely on them. What that relationship entails is a strict duty to put the interests of the beneficiary first, to avoid both the reality and the appearance of a conflict of interests, and to meet the very highest standards of candor and disclosure. It is amazing that no advocate has sought to bring the doctor-patient relationship within the fiduciary concept. It would seem to fit like a glove.

I suppose my audience is astute enough to see how appropriate the explicit imposition of fiduciary responsibilities on the doctor-patient or doctor-experimental subject relationship would be. I hope this makes my initial point that, special situations apart, there is nothing in the newly fashioned regulations that goes further or is more sensitive to the substance of morality than these ancient legal concepts.

Whatever the reasons, the innovation and amelioration that the regulations represent are not at all in the direction of substantive innovation. Rather, what the regulations do and have done splendidly is to force previous attention to these traditional safeguards. These regulations force the building of a record prior to undertaking the experiment. In this way, the kind of after-the-fact rationalization and fudging of what actually took place will not occur. In short, the reform is not a reform in the substance of what decency, fairness, and fidelity to professional standards require. It is an administrative reform making more visible the often invisible decisions so that the ancient substantive standards may be applied to them.

Now let us come to the problem of fetal research, which is simply the most vexed and difficult of the special category of problems that the Commission is dealing with. There are two extreme positions, both of which seem to me plainly unacceptable as a basis for a national consensus.

One of them would say that the fetus until the moment of a normal birth is simply a piece of the mother's body to which anything at all may happen so long as she consents to it. In other words, there are those who would say that fetal research at all stages presents no moral problems whatsoever.

The other extreme position is the notion that a fetus is a person from the moment of conception, and therefore from that moment has all the rights of any other person. Thus, for instance, its informed consent must be obtained prior to any experimentation. I do not mean to say that this latter extreme position can be shown to be wrong; it

cannot. It cannot, however, be shown to be right. And where a position such as that of fetal humanity from the moment of conception is
totally unacceptable to the moral intuitions of a substantial and
respectable body of decent citizins, it is incumbent on those who urge
this position to demonstrate it, and to demonstrate it on the basis of
premises and forms of reasoning acceptable and understandable to all
reasonable persons, not just to those subscribing to special sectarian
positions. These are the extremes.

How, then, is the Commission to discharge its obligation? What the
prior experience or the success of the federal guidelines and regulations suggest is the following: It is unreasonable, unhistorical -- I
would say fatuous -- to expect a central bureaucracy or a national commission to produce substantive wisdom in this area. It is unreasonable
to expect the Commission to resolve in four months a centuries-old
problem of deep philosophical controversy.

What can the Commission do? It must recognize its limitations. It
must recognize that it is a political commission expected to reach a
practical resolution to the theoretical problem that it cannot resolve.
The Commission must realize that if they embrace either extreme, their
resolution cannot command respect. Since they cannot possibly come up
with adequate justification for embracing either extreme position, a
decision at either extreme must appear as brute, political fiat.

What is expected of the Commission must be practical wisdom, and in
this area practical wisdom must recognize the diversity of views and the
evolving nature of the moral sensibilities involved. Just as the HEW
in proposing regulations for general research did not seek to develop
new substantive standards, but had recourse to the traditions of decency
in the community as a whole, so here, I think, that what the Commission
can do is to allow those community judgments of decency to have an impact on the practice of research. Concretely this means bringing
things out into the open, making considerations explicit, forcing justification, exposing practices and protocols to criticism and judgment.
There should not be laws, however, enshrining either extreme position.
There should not be prosecutions, firings, and reprisals based on either
extreme position, because none of this is justified by the state of the
arguments that can be made in the secular, pluralistic society. The
best that the Commission can do is to allow the variegated moral consciousness of the many people in this country to work on this issue, to
work on it candidly, openly, and with sound information. No more is
wise, no more is justified.

MAURICE HILLEMAN

The planet Earth has always been a very unsafe place. Plagues, pesti-
lence, epidemics, and pandemics have swept across the world populations,
and these have been augmented by mass migrations of peoples, by poor
socioeconomic conditions, and by wars. Preventive medicine has helped
make the world less unsafe. My own career has been in this field,

largely in vaccine development and evaluation, and it is in that context that I speak today.

As all of us know, the revolutionary discoveries by Robert Koch and Louis Pasteur led to understandings of the cause of infectious diseases, their mode of transmission, the means for interrupting contagion, and the methods for making prophylactic vaccines -- understandings that have provided the basis for modern preventive medicine. In fact, the dramatic lengthening of the average human lifespan to the biblical three score and ten years derives largely from the benefits of preventive medicine. This accomplishment that we now take for granted rests heavily upon years of experimentation, which included studies carried out in man himself. It is vital, I think, that such studies be continued to permit the development of new vaccines and preventive measures. In no field of human endeavor can so much good be accomplished with so little risk during the developmental stages.

I assume that no one would argue seriously that study of promising new vaccines in man should stop. The epicenter of the present debate is really not whether, but how to proceed, with what protections for the patient and constraints on the investigator and his institution. There have been occasional excesses of zeal and bad judgment in formulating and conducting human trials in the past. This has led to growing concern over the ethical aspects of human experimentation, and to consideration and enactment of ways to control it by means of legislative and regulatory processes. Clearly, balanced laws and reasonable regulation can contribute to progress provided that they remove and prevent the bad and that they promote the good within a framework of what is feasible and what is proper. Draconian measures, however, are not needed. Society must countenance some risk in order to achieve benefits.

There is a particularly favorable benefit-to-risk ratio in the study of new vaccines. Much knowledge can be gained with little risk to the human subject. A vaccine is a biological substance, either living or dead, that with acceptable or even sometimes no clinical side effects imparts worthwhile immunity against an infectious disease. It may be made and it may be administered in different ways. But the important factor is that it must induce immune responses in the host, measured both serologically and in terms of prevention of disease, and that the clinical side effects be well tolerated or nonexistent. The preparation of modern vaccines rests on a century of technology and precedent that permits the making of preparations for which safety and efficacy can be assured with a high level of certainty, although seasoned judgment is still a necessary ingredient.

The clinical tests of new vaccines are initiated only after the chemical, physical, and biological attributes of the product have been exhaustively defined. First tests in human beings are always restricted to small numbers, and their main purpose is to detect possible clinical reactions and to measure antibody responses. Numbers of individuals given the vaccine are gradually expanded, consistent with demonstrated safety and immune responses in the previous tests. Finally, there is

193

expansion to large numbers of persons to measure protective efficacy
against the natural disease in properly controlled studies and to
assure safety under conditions of large-scale use.

Necessary to the accomplishment of these objectives is the collection
of several samples of patients' blood by venipuncture for serologic
testing, the examination of the subject in the process of making clinical observations, and the inclusion in controlled studies of persons
in the control group who receive something other than the vaccine under
test. In these studies it is common practice, insofar as possible, to
give the people in the control group a different vaccine that they need
anyway, and to offer the test vaccine to the controls at such time as
the study is terminated, so that they, too, may enjoy the benefits that
the vaccine affords.

In testing vaccines it is necessary to select study subjects who have
not had previous experience with the agent in nature, and hence are not
already immune to it. For most infectious diseases, this means children of young age, although some vaccines are directed against diseases
that affect adults as well. The question naturally arises as to the
considerations and criteria that govern the selection of study patients,
both children and adults. One principle we have followed is that laid
down by the late Dr. Joseph Stokes, who said, in effect, that all possible safeguards must be taken to guarantee the safety of the vaccine
being given and that the vaccine must be of potential benefit to the
subject himself. In the choice of subjects, it has proved most desirable to include persons in institutions as well as those of open populations. Persons in institutions, such as military establishments,
prisons, or special facilities for handicapped children, such as the
mentally retarded, often provide the best circumstances for study of a
new preventive agent, since large numbers of the persons still susceptible to a particular disease may be present in a sequestered environment. The opportunity for close observation and supervision makes it
readily possible to ascertain whether any clinical reaction occurs.
The persons who are given the vaccine may receive its benefits far in
advance of the time when the vaccine becomes generally available. There
may also be special advantage to the handicapped, since their infectious diseases often are more severe than in normal persons and such
illness may add to the afflictions from which these persons are already
suffering. The inclusion of institutionalized volunteers in clinical
studies assures the availability of subjects in a single location where
continuing surveillance can be assured. The volunteer, in return, has
the benefit of the protection afforded by the vaccine and, in addition,
the opportunity to contribute to a most useful endeavor that will give
him personal satisfaction. This is especially true of prison
volunteers.

The ethical judgment in vaccine studies involving children and adults
in open and in sequestered situations seems to weigh heavily on the side
of doing such studies under proper safeguards. The potential benefit
to the individual and to society is high, and the risk and inconvenience
to the individual is low. The necessary inclusion of such low-risk

194

procedures as venipuncture, the need for controls who do not actually
receive the vaccine under test, and the ordinary obligations of physician to patient, all suggest the essentiality of providing full information to study patients, and in the case of children, to their parents
and/or their guardians. It is a reasonable requirement that studies to
be carried out be reviewed in advance by groups qualified to assess the
medical and scientific factors involved, and also to assess the studies
from the patients' point of view. But deprivation of the opportunity
to carry out proper studies that would lead to progress toward better
health carries its own burden and may, indeed, be unethical, if not
immoral, in itself.

All clinical studies of vaccine are carried out under laws and regulations that include informed written consent, institutional review
committee concurrence, and review by the Bureau of Biologics of the
U.S. Food and Drug Administration. For the most part these controls
function well and do not prevent the conduct of clinical research in
the United States, although they may slow the process markedly and may
even prevent the conduct of studies in some countries.

Let me mention some of contributions that recently developed vaccines
have made to society. Measles virus vaccine was first introduced in
1963 and has now been given to more than 69 million persons in the
United States. The Center for Disease Control has estimated that the
vaccine in the first ten years of use has saved 2,400 lives, has aver-
ted 7,900 cases of mental retardation, and has yielded a net economic
saving of $1.3 billion. Live mumps virus vaccine, introduced in 1967,
has now been given to more than 19 million persons and has led to reduction of mumps to very low level, resulting in dramatic reduction in
mumps encephalitis and death. Live rubella virus vaccine was introduced in 1969 and has now been given to more than 53 million persons
in the United States. Congenital rubella syndrome has been reduced
about twentyfold, and the large-scale epidemic predicted for the early
1970s, that might have caused 20,000 fetal deaths and 30,000 cases of
congenital damage, as it did in 1964, has not materialized. The new
meningococcus vaccine affords high levels of protection against meningococcal meningitis that is currently epidemic in Brazil and in other
nations.

If you look to the future, vaccines against human hepatitis, pneumococcal pneumonia, cytomegalovirus-induced mental retardation, and
chicken pox, as well as vaccines against syphilis, gonorrhea and other
acute infectious diseases, seem clearly on the horizon. Cancer in man
gives evidence of viral involvement, and here too, important vaccine
probes are being carried out. Ultimately, the huge reservoir of chronic
degenerative diseases -- which may be due in large measure to the rav-
ages of ordinary viruses in extraodinary circumstance, and to viruses
as yet undefined or undiscovered -- may yield to preventive approaches.
Viral diseases are preventable, and the eventual control of the as yet
uncontrolled diseases offers a huge magnitude of benefit for mankind
that can further extend man's productive lifespan and, more importantly,
help assure his health and well-being during his childhood, youth,

young adulthood, and maturity. Achievement of such goals depends on our capacity to study new agents in human populations.

A great deal of attention is focused today, and quite properly so, on the moral and the ethical aspects of studies that have been, are being, or will be conducted, with particular emphasis on the implications of such studies for the subject. I hope that the same degree of attention can also be focused on the moral and ethical aspects of the inability of qualified investigators to conduct sound studies under proper auspices and agreed upon controls. It seems to me that the other side of the coin is not being sufficiently examined. If we agree that progress in human health is worthwhile, if we agree that testing new products in man is necessary before their widespread use, then it seems to me we must also agree that it is unethical and immoral -- to use terms frequently heard at this Forum -- for society, either through its legislative, regulatory, and judicial processes, or through the infinitely more powerful force of public opinion, to impose unnecessary constraints and restraints so that testing cannot be carried out at all. And it seems equally unethical and immoral for segments of our society, be they institutions, states, or whatever, to declare themselves off limits for all such testing, counting on the fact that someone else, somewhere, here or abroad, will participate and that they will then benefit without having shared in whatever slight risk might have been involved in the testing process.

I feel optimistic that the good judgment of everyone involved in the decision-making equation -- and the participants and discussants here today are representative of that group -- will cut through this current complexity and provide standards and procedures that will promote rather than hinder clinical research in man. It is in the nature of man to seek and find ways to give his children and succeeding generations a richer and more beneficial heritage than he himself received from the generations that preceded him. I trust this Forum will lead us in that affirmative direction.

RICHARD MERRILL

I would like to enlarge the range of debate and dialogue and dilemma that the proceedings of the past day and a half have developed for us by introducing a factor that has been alluded to but not really examined: the processes by which government agencies become involved and intervene in the decision-making processes of investigators and subjects.

Most of the discussion so far has centered on what should be the criteria for human experimentation, for selection, for exclusion, for admission, for development. I want to examine briefly the responsibilities of one government agency, the Food and Drug Administration, with major responsibility in the area of human investigation, and suggest some of the additional problems that have to be addressed and have to be confronted when we decide what sorts of standards ought to be applied. Let me enter a caveat at the outset. As a teacher of administrative law I view myself as an observer of growing federal intervention in this area, not as an advocate. I say this, knowing full well that that distinction is going to be lost in the course of the discussion, but it is important to make it now.

The structure of my remarks somewhat resembles the story that Dr. Eisenberg told us yesterday about Moses and his arrival at the Red Sea -- the good news and the bad news. Except that my remarks, it seems to me, have the particular virtue of being interpreted in either way. The message comes in two parts. The Food and Drug Administration has this enormous potential authority to regulate and protect human experimentation with new drugs. The other part of the news is that sometimes that system doesn't work very well, and there are enormous limitations on the power of that agency to protect those interests.

The dialogue the past two days has suggested how very difficult are the ethical issues that are involved in trying to develop standards for human experimentation. The competing values between the individual's rights to bodily integrity and society's desire for greater knowledge, and sometimes the physician-investigator's obligation to preserve life, come into clash whenever we try to develop the substantive guidelines for human experimentation. And this listing vastly oversimplifies the values that compete in even the simple cases. When you introduce the further question of what should be the role of government in monitoring the observance and development of the standards that we through consensus or through some political processes agree should be observed, the clash of interest becomes even more complex and the problems of identifying the questions to be answered, much less answering them, becomes more difficult.

The role of the U.S. Food and Drug Administration, which is the focus of my remarks, it seems to me provides an example of this additional complexity. Government regulation of drug testing also exposes a range of issues, issues essentially of a process or an enforcement kind that seem to me to lie outside the main center of the National Commission mandate and are not likely to receive the major force of its attention.

In the areas to which the FDA's jurisdiction extends, the Federal Food, Drug, and Cosmetic Act gives it plenary authority to prescribe any standards for the conduct of clinical investigations of new drugs that can be said to "relate to the protection of the public health." A very broad statutory standard indeed. And thus, although the formal relationship between the National Commission and the responsibilities of the Food and Drug Administration is somewhat murky, it is probably quite true, as Charles Halpern suggested yesterday, that the FDA currently has the statutory authority to embody in regulations and require the observance of any ethical standard that the Commission discerned and announced.

The FDA has already imposed a number of important requirements for the conduct of clinical investigations of new drugs designed for the protection of human subjects, and most of you are familiar with many of them. A manufacturer must conduct preclinical tests in animals before a drug can be given to a human being. And before commencing human testing, he must submit a testing program and allow the FDA a month in which to examine it and suggest changes or prohibit going forward with the investigational program. The sponsoring manufacturer must obtain from each investigator a written commitment that the testing will be conducted under his personal supervision and that informed consent will be obtained in writing from all experimental subjects and, except in "exceptional cases," from all persons receiving the drug for treatment.

If a study is to be conducted in an institutional setting, the FDA regulations require the prior approval of the institutional review committee. Both investigators and the sponsoring manufacturer are required to maintain detailed test records, open to FDA inspection, and the sponsor must submit immediately to the agency all alarming findings of adverse reactions or side effects.

These are not requirements that reflect indifference to the well-being of human subjects. Undoubtedly, the substantive standards that the FDA requires be observed are going to require some strengthening, perhaps some clarification, perhaps even some dramatic revision as a result of the work of the National Commission and other further public deliberations in this area in the future. So, for example, if there is consensus achieved on the question of the status of children, on the status of prisoners, on the status of other groups whose capacity for voluntary informed consent is to be questioned, the FDA is presently empowered under the present statute, and could be disposed to embody those new requirements in regulations formally required to be observed.

But now the rub: higher legal standards alone, it seems to me, will not assure full protection for human subjects. The difficult problems in protecting human subjects are not simply the problems of agreeing on what should be the guidelines on the conduct of the research but they are problems as well of control, of jurisdiction, and enforcement and final assignment of responsibilities.

Let me give you some examples of ways in which, under the present law, responsibility falls through the crack or, at least, responsibility of the government agency ostensibly bearing the congressional mandate is limited or severely constricted.

The Food and Drug Administration currently has no authority to regulate human experimentation with medical devices or with cosmetics or food. The present law gives the agency control only over investigational uses of new drugs. While the agency has occasionally been quite ingenious in extending the definition of drug to embrace items that you and I might on a quick glance conclude were devices or something other than drugs, the fact that it has resorted to this in order to assure the protection of preclinical testing to the eventual consumers of products like that is simply a dramatic indication of the limits on its practical jurisdiction.

Secondly, as Secretary Weinberger intimated in his comments, the FDA lacks authority over clinical investigations conducted with drugs that don't move in interstate commerce. Now this is not a severe practical limitation on the FDA's authority, but it underlies one that is, one that has been alluded to before and was the subject of considerable attention before Senator Kennedy's subcommittee, whose deliberations were instrumental in part in the creation of a national commission. Because the FDA's jurisdiction is tied to the interstate movement of a drug, the status of a drug, as mislabled or misbranded or experimental, depends upon its condition when it crosses a state line. So, for example, if I ship from Charlottesville, Virginia to Seattle, Washington a drug that has been approved by the FDA for use solely in adults, it is lawful when it passes the state lines in between those two jurisdictions so long as it bears labeling indicating its appropriate use and limitations on that appropriate use. When it reaches Seattle, the physician there can lawfully prescribe that drug for the treatment of that condition or for any other condition without violating any other regulation or any statute administered by the Food and Drug Administration. The same would hold true for the pharmacy that agrees to fill that prescription. This can be true even if the use is one that the FDA has evaluated and rejected, as well as if it is one which the FDA simply has not had brought to its attention.

When the Seattle physician prescribes that drug for several patients or several Seattle physicians prescribe it for one or more of the individual patients for the unapproved use, we have a situation that can fairly be characterized, it seems to me, as experimental. But it is one, nonetheless, over which the Food and Drug Administration has no effective control to assure the observance of whatever standards are agreed upon for the protection of the human subject. That experimental use of a drug approved by the FDA greatly alarmed the Senate Subcommittee investigating the human experimentation in the United States, particularly in the context of drugs DES and Depro-Provera. The description "experimental" is the FDA's and the Senate Subcommittee's. Others would describe what happens when the Seattle physician prescribes that drug for a new use or a new condition outside the bounds of the FDA evaluated and approved labeling as simply his exercise of reasonable judgment in the interest of treating his patient. These two divergent characterizations of the same event suggest the nature of the values that conflict here.

Perhaps the most serious limitation on the FDA's practical ability to ensure observance of ethical standards in clinical trials lies in its remoteness from clinical investigators. The Food and Drug Act imposes obligations -- to conduct preclinical tests, to obtain assurances of supervision, to obtain informed consent, and to make reports -- on "the manufacturer or sponsor" of the investigation, not on the investigator. Indeed, one provision of the Food and Drug Act bespeaks a conscious congressional intention to limit the FDA's ability to deal directly with investigators where it provides: "Nothing in this subsection shall be construed to require any clinical investigator to submit directly to the Secretary reports on the investigational use of drugs." Accordingly the FDA relies primarily on sponsors of drug tests to assure them that they are properly conducted. I have no doubt that most sponsors take that obligation very seriously.

To be sure, the agency can, through procedures established by regulations, suspend the right of an investigator to receive investigational
drugs that move in interstate commerce, and has done so on about two
dozen different occasions. And it does require sponsors to demand from
their investigators a written and signed commitment to maintain proper
records, obtain informed consent, and permit FDA inspection of their
records. But the hard facts are that the FDA lacks both the manpower
and the legal authority to monitor clinical investigators closely, and
to assure faithful observance of its substantive standards.

The conduct of clinical trials of new drugs is a collaborative and,
hopefully in most instances, a cooperative undertaking among the FDA,
the drug manufacturers and test sponsors, individual investigators, and
institutional review committees. But one should not be surprised, given
the rather odd framework of regulation here, that sometimes the process
doesn't work altogether. And we might well conclude that full protection of the rights of human subjects of clinical investigations of new
drugs is going to require some revision or enlargement of FDA authority,
as well as resources, over the conduct of those tests. Whether this is
done or not, it seems clear that we ought to demand some very firm veri-
fication of where the primary responsibility lies for adherence to the
standards that are eventually adopted.

In conclusion let me make two observations. One is triggered by a
comment made twice during the past two days, registering, it seems to
me, a very well-founded concern on the part of individuals or social
groups that drug products reach the market and are widely used before
they have been fully investigated and fully tested in human beings.
The characterization from a member of the audience that women taking
oral contraceptives are human guinea pigs is one that I have no doubt
is very very strongly felt and not wholly unjustified. But there is an
ambivalence to the situation of those who object to experimentation in
the marketplace, which, to some extent, is what goes on with respect to
drugs. This is an invitation, indeed a demand, it seems to me, to do
more investigation in the premarketing clinical setting. If we want to
be sure what the oral contraceptives are going to do, we are going to
have to expose more persons to risks during the premarketing stage --
either that or we are going to do without oral contraceptives. We may
be prepared to forgo some benefits in the area of food additives, where
utility perhaps is not as compelling; but we are not as likely to be
prepared to make that kind of trade-off with respect to drugs that can
provide, as I think most people would agree, very substantial benefits.

Finally, it seems to me that there has been running through the comments of some of the people at this podium an alarm about the fact that
there is a growing public interest and concern about human experimentation. It seems to me that rather than view with alarm the prospect
that the public is going to get involved in and be concerned about how
government agencies, drug manufacturers, clinical investigators undertake and carry out their business and the standards that they observe,
in this day and age we have to be prepared to welcome that, we should

invite it. And I would agree with Dr. Ingelfinger's comment that there is a responsibility, indeed an opportunity, for clinical investigators in the biomedical research community to invite public attention and sell the importance of biomedical research. There is no doubt that this is an important, mandatory, worthwhile undertaking. I don't think we should be afraid of public exposure and public deliberation. We would be unrealistic if we tried to avert it.

INQUIRY AND COMMENTARY

LEWIS THOMAS: I would like to ask the panel if they will wait for a short while before beginning their own discussion until we have heard something from the discussants or members of the audience at large.

DEWITT STETTEN, JR.: I am with the National Institutes of Health. I have failed to hear something that I think should be a part of the equation that is set up when we try to balance risks or costs against benefits. What is the cost or the risk of curbing or constraining the right of free inquiry? Free inquiry is in many ways comparable to free speech or free press, and it is probably only an historical accident that it was not specifically included in the First Amendment. The accident, of course, rests with the fact that James Madison was trained in law, as were many of his playmates at the Constitutional Convention, and lawyers like to talk and they like to write. Had these gentlemen been trained in science, I suspect that free inquiry might perfectly well have been included as one of the guaranteed freedoms.

Free inquiry, like free speech, would be subject to certain limitations; but like free speech, we should relinquish this freedom infrequently and only with a certain amount of agony and only when there is a real and present danger demonstrable if we fail to relinquish it. That there is a cost involved in relinquishing freedom of inquiry has been repeatedly demonstrated in history. This recently was brought to the attention of the televiewing public once again, in Dr. Bronowski's presentation of the life of Galileo, in which it was his interpretation that the judgments of the Inquisition constraining Galileo to abjure from inquiry in certain areas caused the shift from Italy and the Catholic countries as leaders in the scientific renaissance to the Protestant countries of the north, leading to Newton and the great astronomers in the Scandinavian and British countries.

I would like to suggest, then, that among the hazards, among the costs to be included in assessing the cost-benefit analysis of constraining physicians and scientists from doing certain things, must be included this effect upon freedom of inquiry.

WILLIAM VODRA: I am Associate Chief Counsel for Drugs, Food and Drug Administration. I would like to pick up on a few items that Professor Merrill touched on and to point out some important subtle differences in the way we approach regulation of research.

The NIH proposals that have been discussed go to the question of funding, that is, when the federal government gives money to support research. When we go over across the line to FDA regulation, we get into the research that is not funded by the federal government but regulated by it in two ways: the denial of the use of the data for certain things, such as supporting the approval of a drug; and criminal sanctions, that is, the investigator goes to jail if he commits certain violations. We must keep this distinction in mind when we are talking about ethics, because ethics and law do not always coincide. And where there is an ambiguity in ethical issues, as Professor Fried pointed out, we must be careful not to take a flat rule by fiat and say that because we do not approve this for a funding purpose we also do not approve it for a regulatory purpose. There is a subtle distinction between when the federal government funds a project and when it regulates conduct. A question comes up again when you ask how far should the federal government intervene and in what way? Do we intervene by criminal sanctions, by funding sanctions, or whatever? And how do we enforce these things? Because these in turn go back to the risks to which you put the individual investigator -- financial risks, criminal sanctions risks, and so forth.

The second point I would like to touch on is the sanctions available to FDA. I think Professor Merrill outlined several of the limitations on FDA very well. But one he did not mention is what the FDA does when we are faced with a study that is "bad" for ethical reasons or scientific reasons. The hard question is put when the study shows a safety problem. When it shows that the drug is effective, we can always reject it and say, "Go back and do it again properly. This was unethical." But if we find out that the study proved the drug unsafe, can we ethically then reject the data? And if we do accept the data, then have we in essence condoned an unethical study? This is the kind of controversy that FDA faces continuously in looking at bad data reports.

Other sanctions available to the FDA are limited really to the suspension of certain privileges of doing drug studies or to criminal sanctions. There may be other ways that we can go, but right now those are the courses available to FDA.

Finally, what happens if the FDA and the federal government reject certain research projects as unethical and thereby, in essence, export that research to other countries where the standards are different? Can we ethically say that what we will not allow to be done on Americans in the United States is acceptable when done in Africa on Africans? I think that is a very difficult ethical question that should be dealt with in our contemplations.

UNIDENTIFIED: Professor Fried raised the point that the United States
   is an open and pluralistic society and thet the Commission ought to
   avoid the two extremes that he noted or argued are existent with
   respect to fetal research. And then he said -- if I am not mis-
   quoting him -- that we ought to have an open, pluralistic solution
   to the problem of fetal research.

   The problem there is that you have set up the wrong model. You
   have set up a model that is appropriate to policy that can be seen
   out of continuum, such as, for example, minimum wage legislation.
   Should we raise it fifty cents, one dollar, two dollars, three dollars? We can compromise, but if you have policy positions on fetal
   research in which you automatically reject the two extreme positions,
   you make it impossible to satisfy a large group -- and in particular
   a group that claims there should be no experimentation on any fetuses. If you have, as I think, really a dichotomy and not a continuum, then you really can't satisfy a very substantial proportion
   of the population's view on this issue. That, I think, is the
   sticking point. The issue is not a continuum, but a dichotomy,
   and the United States is not very good at dealing with issues in
   which there is a dichotomy, particularly a moral dichotomy.

GERALD GAULL: I am Professor of Pediatrics at Mount Sinai, and I am
   probably one of the few people in this room who has ever dealt with
   a human fetus and who specifically does experiments on the human
   fetus. I do not consider myself a venal man. I do not consider myself a manslaughterer or a grave robber.

   I was very much taken with Professor Fried's presentation and
   the caveats there, because, unlike the last discussant, I do not
   think it is a dichotomy. I have had human fetuses in my hand at all
   stages of development, and I do not know what a "living" human fetus
   is. Therefore, I do not know exactly whether I am complying or not
   complying with the regulations to be promulgated.

   The thing that I liked most in Professor Fried's talk was the fact
   that he recognized the frailty of morality and the necessity for
   tentativeness in our decisions. I am not as certain of the morality
   of what I am doing as those who consider me immoral are about what I
   do. And I would note that 500 years ago those who consider what I
   do to be immoral were absolutely certain that the world was flat and
   that this was the center of the universe.

JAY GOLD: I am Assistant Attorney General for the Commonwealth of Pennsylvania. Dr. Hilleman said that the words *moral* and *ethical* have
   been used a lot at this Forum. Nobody has really gone into them very
   deeply. I think Professor Fried has tried, but I don't think he has
   been successful.

   Professor Fried, you spoke of both community standards of decency
   and of moral intuitions, but in neither case was I really sure what
   you meant. In the one case you said that since the Commission has
   only four months and can't solve all the issues in that time, it

should realize that it is a political creature and should try to limit itself to codifying the standards of decency of the community. You said this right after vehemently castigating the decision in the Edelin trial. The verdict in that decision was rendered by a jury of twelve good men and true, some of whom were women. One might think that verdict, therefore, conforms with the standards of decency of a considerable segment of the community. By your reasoning it is possible that the Commission might not only wind up codifying that decision, but extending its spirit to other areas.

When you spoke about moral intuition, it was in the context that the idea that personhood begins at conception goes against the moral intuitions of a great many people, and that, therefore, the proponents of that idea have the responsibility to prove it on the basis of premises that are acceptable to all reasonable people. It is true, I think, that there are a large number of people to whom the idea that personhood begins at some time other than conception is repugnant to their moral intuition. I don't know whether you would want the responsibility of proving to them that it begins at some other time, especially since you implied very strongly that there was, really, no clear-cut answer to the question. So while I applaud your raising issues that others have evaded here, I am afraid that, ultimately, you wound up doing what F. H. Bradley said philosophy did, which is finding bad reasons for what you believe on instinct.

GEORGE HILL: This is for the Vice President of Merck Sharp & Dohme Research Laboratories. I would like to know whether the research money which is going to be funded is public money and how you expect to spend it? I would like to know your prospectus as to how you intend to analyze the cost-benefits of your endeavor. And I would like to know whether you are prepared to set up a fund for the benefits that your corporation, and medicine in general, will derive.

THOMAS: That is as far as we can take the questions. I will now ask the panel to clarify everything about everything.

FRIED: Well, I think I was asked about why it is that I put the burden of proof on those who suggest that personhood begins at conception. Since I can't say, which I cannot, when personhood begins, why is the burden of proof on me? The answer is quite simple. I am not trying to stop anybody from doing anything. I am not calling anybody a murderer, and I am not trying to call anybody a manslaughterer. Therefore, the burden that rests on me is, I think, somewhat lighter.

MERRILL: The comment directed at free inquiry prompts me to say something I thought about before. I don't like to be defensive of lawyers in this posture, but I suppose I will be. I don't think lawyers are any less committed to free inquiry than people in other disciplines. But it does seem to me that the dialogue of the past

204

two days has suggested a divergence in viewpoint that stems, perhaps, in part from the differences in professional training -- and I speak now simply of the researchers and the lawyers.

Lawyers tend to view their constituencies -- that is, the people for whom they have professional responsibility -- in a much shorter time frame than do researchers. It is in the present, now, and I think our attitude tends to be questioning, skeptical, and negative. We ask "Why".

I think the researchers, quite properly, view their professional responsibility as extending into future generations. That brings us to these issues from somewhat different directions and produces not misunderstanding, because we don't have misunderstanding here, it produces disagreement.

HILLEMAN: Obviously, if a product is developed that is useful to people they will buy it, and there will be a profit. This profit, then, is largely used to go back into developing new things that people need for the future. A certain amount of the profits from many corporations, and I know from our own, goes into a foundation and is used for promotion of medical education, perhaps other things. There are a number of such support type possibilities. I would merely point out that if one becomes too gratuitous with too many benefits, it is only going to raise the price for the consumer.

I would just like to say one other thing. During these two days we have heard a lot of issues raised, and I doubt if this thing went on for a year there would be anything new or significant. My hope would be that one would get on with the resolutions, that we can stop all this discussion, and get on with some sort of a uniform code. Obviously, there are going to be lots of different groups of people who are going to participate. I do hope that those who speak for these people will indeed represent them and that they will have their informed consent, because, very largely, many of the leaders of these vocal groups are representing only the establishment of a particular group, and not necessarily speaking for the total group. So I hope we can just get on with these things in a very reasonable way.

CHARLES LOWE: I would like to invite some more comment from Dr. Fried on one particular aspect of his presentation. In his opening remarks he said that the regulations issued for public comment by the Department invoke established principles rather than plowing new ground, that is, in the legal sense.

On the other hand, in reading the statute that the Congress passed, I cannot help but have a sense that it was the opinion of the Congress that there was, in fact, a need for new legal ground, and that this developed rather directly from the fact that technical advances had occurred for which there was no legal background, particularly, for example, behavioral control, fetal surgery, and perhaps experimentation on minors when it is of no benefit to them.

Would you be kind enough to comment on the perceived need for rather new legal principles rather than falling back on established ones?

FRIED: In respect to those areas, there is a great deal to what you say. That is a qualified remark. I was referring, though, to the regulations that have been passed and that have made an enormous and beneficial difference. Those regulations, I really do think, simply carry forward in an administratively much more potent way established legal principles.

Referring to those new areas of which you spoke, I think there really is a puzzle about those because they don't fit the established categories. But I put it to you that whatever you come up with, whether it is in four months or four years, you are going to proceed on the analogy of the existing concepts that we use. In dealing with psychosurgery, you are going to take something like informed consent and move on from it, because, frankly, I don't know how else you can proceed. I do not believe that new standards will be born like Athene from the brow of Zeus, even though you are not Zeus.

FUTURE
POLICY OPTIONS
AND SUMMARY

FUTURE POLICY OPTIONS AND SUMMARY
_____

The Panel for Inquiry:

Richard E. Behrman
Ivan L. Bennett, Jr.
Douglas D. Bond
Howard H. Hiatt
Frederick C. Robbins
Lewis Thomas

LEWIS THOMAS

The members of the Panel for Inquiry have been present since the beginning of our proceedings. Some of them have been active in other aspects
of the Forum; some have remained relatively quiet. All of them have
sat these long hours, storing up new knowledge and synthesizing new
wisdom. Each of them is now asked to share his views with us.

RICHARD BEHRMAN

I have some general reflections. It seems to me that the arrogance and
the lack of perception of the physician-scientists here about their
activities within the spectrum of general social activities and their
appreciation of the changing moral atmosphere have only been matched --
with the exception of Mr. Fried -- by the idolatry of the lawyers for
the advocacy system to resolve all social problems, and their lack of
effort to understand the decision-making process in the health field
and to suggest appropriate options.
   That has been matched only by the failure of the sociologists to project social options and their implications that can be used for the
basis of decision-making rather than to be content with describing the
trends.
   That is matched only, in my estimation, by the ethicists and philosophers who have been preoccupied with using the current problems as a
forum for propagating and publicizing preexisting absolute ideological
positions, rather than helping to work out new social solutions and
modifying their own underlying assumptions.

Perhaps that has been matched last, but certainly not least, by the pandering to sensationalism of the special interest groups that have preferred to do this rather than to engage in a rational evaluation of the facts and an open evaluation of the issues.

I would like to make two assumptions: That there have been, continue to be, and perhaps always will be some serious abuses in carrying on human investigation; that some research -- on the fetus, on children, on special groups, some of which cannot give independent informed consent -- may be needed for the sake of future generations, even though no direct therapeutic benefit for the individual comes from it.

If we want a system that at least deals with these two tentative assumptions, then the real issue to be dealt with now is what social mechanisms are possible to devise to reconcile these two considerations? To get back to some comments that were made earlier, it is an issue, it seems to me, of balancing different rights and interests, individual and societal. This is similar to what is done in many other medical decision-making processes as well as nonmedical ones in which judgments are made and in which there is no set of rights and wrongs. Free speech vs. public safety is the obvious one that has been alluded to by one of the speakers.

In part, I am disagreeing with what Dr. McDermott brought up yesterday. He said that we institutionalize social decisions when one person's decision may hurt another. I would say that we don't generally do that in our society. We certainly don't in most medical decisions. We allow the people closest to the decision to make errors, even at considerable cost to themselves, their families, and to society. Only in exceptional circumstances do we make the judgment that someone else will make fewer errors if we allow another group to do it. I happen, personally, to think that this area of human activity does require some institutionalization beyond what has existed before. On the other hand, I think it obviously has dangers that have been alluded to by a number of the people on the various panels.

I would like to state briefly a few of the characteristics of the mechanisms that seem to me to be important and to have been emphasized by various people, because these are the building blocks that we have to use to develop some kind of new social mechanisms to deal with this problem.

Certainly, openness has been a recurring theme. I think it is also clear that the predominant influence in making judgments has to rest with those other than the biomedical people, but not exclusive of biomedical people because then we are just espousing getting the least-informed judgments. On the other hand, the nonbiomedical people shouldn't be dominated by special interest groups who are organized for the political process.

Also, we need to be able to redecide at regular intervals. We need to be able to make the judgments again and again, and the institution-alized system that we devise should not be obstructive to allowing us to change those judgments.

We must remember that there really are dangers in the institution-alization, as Dr. Eisenberg pointed out. It is easy in the propensity of bureaucracies to make negative decisions as the safest decisions, and I think that applies within universities, in deans' offices, as well as within the federal government.

I think we need a continuing upgrading of the general level of public understanding of the decision-making process if we are going to modify the system in a rational way.

The conflicts of interest are central: the benefits for the present and the future generation vs. the respect for the individual. I personally don't think they are any more resolved than Dr. Fried does by choosing one or the other of the two extremes. What we need to develop, then, is one set of national guidelines or regulations along the lines that the Commission is considering.

I would like to mention some particulars that might be considered merely as an example of the kind of analysis that should be gone through if we are going to use protection committees. Although I am taking an analogy from the common law, this is not to suggest that a legal process or an administrative law process is the appropriate one to make these decisions. Let us assume that the mechanism we need is some kind of community group to make judgments relevant to the particular areas of concern. I don't think it makes sense for the Commission to specific-cally designate the composition of these groups. It would be much more appropriate in most situations to put out some broad guidelines to make sure that the groups are composed of a wide variety of interests, mainly nonbiomedical. That will be determined very much by the local situa-tion, whether the hospital doing the research is in Harlem or in Bronx-ville, New York. On the other hand, there are certain principles and there may be specific situations for which the details have to be laid out quite concretely.

How are we going to treat the different kinds of institutions? I think it would be appropriate for the Commission to go into that. Look at the different nature of university hospitals vs. community hospitals vs. physician's offices vs. institutions for the retarded. In the university hospitals, for example, a diverse board made up of special interests from the community might be the easiest to set up. In a community hospital, you might have to require some people from outside of the community to be members of those boards. In the case of insti-tutions, particularly isolated ones like those for prisoners or for the mentally retarded, the very specific composition of outside groups should be designated for whole regions and should be required to be approved centrally.

General guidelines about the administrative process certainly are needed. Some of those have been already mentioned, and they are needed to ensure the openness and the candidness of the procedure.

It seems to me that informed consent has to be defined broadly enough to include substitute consent. Unless it is, we eliminate at all the possibility that at some point we may want to do nontherapeutic

212

research on a subgroup because there is such a substantial benefit for that subgroup and a relatively small risk that we want to be able to make that social decision. How we apply that doctrine of substitute consent and exactly what it consists of I certainly, at this point, couldn't speculate. But I know one thing: it can't be an absolute doctrine. It has got to be able to include the poor, the fetus, and the child under certain circumstances.

Somehow we have to develop some concept for nontherapeutic research, but possibly also for therapeutic research that deals with the reasonable likelihood of a substantial benefit relative to the nature of the risks incurred. Even though that is not precise, it is precise enough for a group of reasonable people to begin to make instance by instance judgments about whether or not a given area of research should be allowed to take place in society.

IVAN BENNETT

I would like to begin with a quotation that James Reston had in his column recently quoting E. B. White: "Most of the special matters people now discuss are pressing, but taken singly or added together do not point in a steady direction that gets me up in the morning to pull on my marching boots."

I would like to try to describe for you what I think I have gotten out of the discussions for the past two days. It is hard for me to say that I got all of this just from the discussions. But it seems to me that the trend in this area where for quite some time now we have been examining policies for clinical investigations -- that is, research using human beings -- points to some very important considerations for which we require more information.

To begin with, I think we need to pay more attention than we have to the composition of the groups from which most volunteers have come. The fact is that a great deal of work has been done with prisoners and with individuals who, for the sake of this Forum, have been described as the poor, but who, as Dr. Ingelfinger has pointed out, are administratively available simply because of the structure of the system in which they receive their care or in which they live. It seems to me that we really do need to enlarge our knowledge and analyze the reasons that, with certain exceptions, volunteers have been drawn from rather selected segments of our society.

The issue of informed consent, which has been raised from time to time during this meeting, is one that we need to understand considerably better. Despite the arguments that I have heard, I remain unconvinced that it is not possible to obtain informed consent from individuals who are institutionalized and who are competent. I think that they are capable of understanding and that they certainly are capable of volunteering. Despite the recognized deficiencies, for example, in our penal system, I do not think that we will advance research or solve many of the problems with that system if we simply decide to remove or narrow the range of options available to these individuals by making it impossible for them to volunteer to participate in studies, whatever their motivations.

Along those lines, one of the things we need to know more about -- and it is obvious that a few efforts have been made in this direction -- is what the impact on the individual or on the group is of participation in one of these volunteer studies. The recent publication of the study done in Somers State Prison takes a step in that direction. It seems to me that the more we know about what the actual impact on the individual, his self-perception, his motivations, and so forth, as a result of participation in one of these studies, the better position we will be in to make selections or set up guidelines for the selection of volunteers.

There are really two problems in terms of the information that is provided to potential volunteers. One of these appears to be the incompleteness of the information that was supplied in certain instances. The incompleteness occurs, perhaps, because of the urgency of time or the amount of effort it would take to provide complete information. It seems obvious, in certain instances, that information has been deliberately withheld, and I know of no one who would consider that to be justified. But I do believe that we need to study very much the information part of informed consent.

Here again it seems to me that it would be quite useful if more of us engaged in the type of study that was done at Somers or in one of the collaborative studies that Dr. Lasagna did in which, after a lapse of time, one went back to the volunteers to see how much of the information that one thought one was transmitting had, in actual fact, been retained. If one can detect a pattern, it seems to me that this would go a long way to providing a basis for improving this communication and understanding. This is an area in which it is possible to increase our knowledge and understanding by a relatively simple effort.

I personally got a great deal from the discussion by Dr. Katz of the ambiguity of motivations that are involved in the transactions that take place not only in the usual physician-patient relationship, but in the relationship between an investigator and volunteers. The more we can clarify our thinking about these ambiguities as they now exist, the more we can clarify our thinking about the motivations of the subject, as well as the motivations of the investigator, we will be in a much better position to understand what some of the dynamics are. In urging that we analyze and identify these things, I am not sure how they can be carried forward, because that is not my field. But I am sure that there are mechanisms that would make it possible for us to better understand the mix of motivations involved.

I am absolutely convinced that in many instances those of us in the medical profession have forgotten or do not bring to the surface of our consciousness what the transaction is that takes place between a physician and a patient, or even between a physician and a member of the public with whom he discussed medical matters. This is something that we need to have in our consciousness. We need to understand better, like it or not, that we speak from a special position, that most people listen to us in a very special way, and that this puts on us a very special responsibility.

The presentation by Dr. Fried was very valuable to me. He was able to put in a framework of principles of law that have existed for a long time what the real purposes of the regulations and guidelines are. He has given me a basis for thinking of this that had not been clarified for me before.

The last point that I would like to touch on has to do with what the mechanisms might be for monitoring on-going research to see to it that the protocols that have been reviewed and approved are actually being implemented, and to see to it that if some unexpected occurrence turns up in the course of a study it will be modified accordingly.

The difficulty that we face to begin with is the enormous size, as Dr. Chalkley has pointed out to us, of the undertaking as it goes on in this country. I see no possible mechanism at the present time except an institutional one by which the institution, through an appropriate organization, probably a committee, would have to monitor the activities going on in the institution. It might be the same committee that presently functions to approve protocols; or a different committee might be required, because it is a very time-consuming endeavor, particularly in an institution of any size.

So far as the composition of the committee is concerned, I know of no institution that objects to the inclusion of individuals who are not primarily engaged in biomedical research. On the other hand, as I say, it is a very time-consuming endeavor. From a practical viewpoint, up until now it has been relatively difficult to obtain individuals from other fields, particularly outside of the institution, who can find the time and effort to devote to this kind of endeavor, no matter how interested they are. Perhaps, as these issues are highlighted in this Forum, there may be more general realization of the importance of discharging this responsibility.

One of the most useful suggestions, which was not first made here but which was repeated here, would be to develop a mechanism for the exchange of experience and information among the committees in this country that have taken on these institutional responsibilities. I would have to say that my attention has been drawn to the fact that certain protocols have been approved in other institutions in New York that our own committee would not have approved. This does not necessarily mean that one was wrong and the other was right. But I do know that it would be useful if the committees could get together to discuss the difference in viewpoints that led to a situation in which a protocol might be approved in one institution while the committee in another institution state flatly that they would never have approved that protocol.

I am sure that in an area like New York City this would be relatively easy. Although it certainly would not be very easy to arrange for some sort of informal exchange on a regular basis among the committees in the New York City area, I would hope that some mechanism could be found

215

so that, whether or not one documents all decisions that are made,
selected decisions that represent the resolution of a particularly
difficult issue might be encapsulated or epitomized in some way so that
this information could become more generally available.

Despite the motivation for discovery or to be first, and so on, I
believe that this type of information could be made available without
encroaching on the privacy of the ideas of the investigators who had
originally proposed the research. I would hope that one practical outcome of this Forum might be that we would find some way in which to
institutionalize the exchange of appropriate information about decisions
that are made in the area of human experimentation and protocols of informed consent.

All in all, I think that this has been a useful conference. It certainly has not found answers to some of the hard questions that must be
faced up to. But it seems to me that it may set the stage for developing mechanisms whereby some of these issues might be resolved to the
satisfaction of not all but of most of us who are concerned, including
the investigators, including the subjects, and including the many other
individuals who quite rightly have begun to question the system as it
has existed in the past.

DOUGLAS BOND

About 1950 a French author, Vercors, wrote a story entitled "You Shall
Know Them" in which a group of missing links is found who resemble
humans remarkably, are gentle, tractable, and highly educable. Soon
they are being used widely to do all sorts of labor. The hero becomes
upset at this exploitation and decides to kill a young one to settle the
issue as to whether or not the creatures are human. The story builds
to a trial in which attempts are made to use anthropological and behavioral criteria to differentiate man from his lower cousins. None
prove satisfactory. If the hero is to win his goal, he will be con-
victed of murder; if he loses, his protégés will be destined for exploitation. The resolution comes when it is decided that the creatures
are indeed human. However, the judge points out that the hero really
slaughtered an animal, since the only criterion for judging humanness
is the acceptance by other humans, and until that was done the creatures were not humans.

This story came to me while listening to the discussions of the last
two days as to when human life begins in the fetus, and as to what
groups of people might be used for testing and other forms of clinical
investigation.

To take the fetus first, some discussion took place as to when it
could be called a person. Hope was expressed that someday we would
know the beginning of life. I doubt very much that we can know the
beginning of life. It will always be a question of our definition.
Life seems to be an even flowing stream, moving from one cell to another, from one life to another; to sample some water from a stream and

216

say "this is the beginning" makes little sense. We need not ponder
the imponderable. There are plenty of other things to do. Arbitrary
decisions in practical matters are good enough. The Supreme Court made
such a judgment when it said, in effect, that a fetus becomes an infant
when it can survive outside the mother's body. Everyone knows it cannot really be independent. The human infant's helplessness demands care
and feeding of the most devoted sort or it will die; but it exits from
the mother's body, and with care it can survive. There is no real
scientific definition here, it's only practical and very useful. Some
other time may someday be chosen, but no matter.

The term "fetal rights" seems unfortunate to me. Everyone is competing for special rights these days, and I hate to get the fetus into
it, although it would be less clamorous than others. The fetus certainly does not know it has rights, and to use such a term borders on
the absurd. Does an ovum have a right to be fertilized? A sperm to
keep its tail? If the point is to respect living tissue, why not just
say so. If one wants to insist on the rights issue, why not follow
the Supreme Court and say that rights begin at their arbitrary line?

Informed consent, now asked for when human beings submit themselves
to medical procedures or when they become subjects in clinical investigations, seems to me to have not only the function of informing the
patient or subject, but also to say to the physician or investigator,
"This is a human being like yourself." It should be a reminder and a
caution.

We humans have a spectrum of humanness in our minds. Those different
from us seem a little less human. In days gone by the poor were less
human. Somehow they didn't feel the same as the more fortunate. The
Calvinist doctrine reinforced the idea that God rewarded the righteous
and promptly, so the unrewarded poor became the unrighteous. The first
prison to be constructed in England in lieu of various maiming punish-
ments was Bridewell House in 1553, dedicated to the "detention and
reformation of the poor."

We are now going through a process of admitting more people to full
humanness: the poor, people of different colors, women, and children.
Where informed consent should have its greatest meaning to the investigator, therefore, should be in those areas where the subject seems
most different. When it comes to the subject, trust in the benevolence
of the investigator must come first. Our discussion to date has centered on imparting sufficient knowledge. But going into scientific
detail on the trial of a new drug whose action is not fully known can
hardly be the main point.

I recently underwent a major operation upon my heart. The surgeon
explained how he would take the mammillary artery and jump a block in
one of my coronaries. Incidentally, he forgot to mention that he would
open my chest. He told me of the overall mortality figures and assured
me that his figures were better. I quickly assented. My wife walked
in at this point and slowed the procedure down. She asked if she could
call on an old friend, Howard Burchell, a cardiologist of note. The
surgeon agreed. Howard called the various physicians and told my wife

"go ahead." She was entirely content. What one wants at such a time
is no detailed explanation, which could be endless, but a competent
and trustworthy synthesis.

Medicine has had a great record in caring for the poor, unmatched by
any profession except the ministry. That the poor in effect paid for
their care by aiding young physicians to learn and by being subjects
for various clinical trials was and is by no means all bad. The supervision of that care has assured a level of scientific care that many
private patients lack. Certainly the poorer patients in the great
teaching hospitals of this country were the first to benefit from the
antibiotics, the various sulfonamides, and new surgical interventions.
But the record is not spotless. Investigators have from time to time
jumped the gun by going too quickly to clinical trial before adequate
animal testing and have in addition practiced poor science. The more
recent controls begun in institutions doing clinical investigation have
done much to curtail careless or thoughtless work. The natural adver-
sarial relationship among investigators is a great safeguard when research is open to scrutiny.

There is a move afoot to include either lawyers or laymen on such
committees. I seriously question this move. Physicians are as a
whole not devoid of humanity, nor are they only cold and detached when
it comes to people or patients. That some may be caught in a private
ambition or in an unwarranted enthusiasm is certainly true, but scrutiny
by colleagues is, for me, the best safeguard. After all, the legal
profession can hardly afford to be righteous at this time.

Investigation is hard work. Nature holds her secrets dear. The
long, tedious, frustrating labor that is the forerunner of a result is
normally hidden. The demands of focusing one's energies in a narrow
band necessitates a kind of tunnel vision that the scientific method
was developed to defend against. Good controls have ruined countless
good findings. Informed consent is another safeguard for the subject.

I would hope that we would not rush to control to the point that
clinical investigation becomes so overburdened with external restraints
that we give up. It is coming dangerously close to that point now. I
am not a clinical investigator in any sense that has been used at this
Forum, so I am happy to speak to it. Mr. Halpern suggested that the
lawyers and the investigators work together to evolve a series of procedures. That is fine with me as long as we do not apply restraint
too quickly and we gather, over time, a decent data base that we can
use to develop policy. At this point there is none. It is characteristic of the law to take one case and derive principle from it.
Science is more inclined to develop a series of cases to derive its
findings. In this instance, I side with the scientists.

HOWARD HIATT

It is difficult to come at the end of two days, at the end of a series
of such thoughtful people, and do much more than just repeat or

underline those things that perhaps need emphasis. That will be largely
what I will do.

Medicine has become an increasingly complicated area, as has clinical
research. Technologic advances, advances in medical capabilities,
changes in our ethics, in our moral outlooks, in our attitudes toward
various groups in our society -- women, consumers -- all of these have
undergone rapid transformations that are still accelerating. But there
has been no concomitant change in the decision-making process in medicine and in medical research; that, to a large extent, is what this
Forum has been about.

Many of the changes that people are seeking really will depend, in
my view, on changes in the practice of medicine and in our health system, as several people have outlined. For example, I think that everybody needs a Howard Burchell. That is what people have been saying to
us. It is not the investigator that can rightly ask informed consent
of the patient. Every patient must have his or her own doctor or some
other person. It can be a social worker, a nurse-practitioner, or
anyone else, but it must be an informed person to whom the individual
can turn for advice as to the reasonableness of his or her own participation in the experiment in question. It is unfair to ask of the
investigator that he attempt to elicit informed consent; it is unfair
to ask of the patient that he give informed consent in the absence of
an ombudsman.

We need a health care system in which there is better data collection. We are doing experiments now and projecting experiments for the
future to answer questions that should reasonably have been answered
long ago. For example, we began giving anticoagulants for a variety of
diseases in the middle '40s. The imprecision of our mechanism of administration of treatment and of our data collection have led us now to
still having unanswered some of the same questions that medical students and physicians and investigators were asking twenty-five years
ago.

Obviously, the conflicts that have been described between the
interests of society and the interests of the individual are going to
be difficult to resolve and will continue to be difficult to resolve.
We did not talk much about the various factors that go into the equation. Surely no research is ethical in which the question being asked
is not a reasonable one; no research is ethical in which the methods
being used are not likely to obtain the results that are sought. Thus,
the evaluation of the question, the evaluation of methodology is as
important in looking at the ethics of a question as are several of the
other factors to which we have referred.

We have not talked enough about the obligations society incurs for
the individuals who participate in research projects. But those are
very real, and they should be and must be codified.

It is clear that all of our considerations are fluid ones. Our
knowledge, our capabilities, our attitudes are changing. What is acceptable in 1975 hopefully will not be acceptable in 1980. Thus, whatever mechanisms we settle upon as satisfactory for looking at today's

problems ought to be continuing ones, mechanisms that permit us to look
on a continuing basis at the changes that inevitably, hopefully, will
be going on.

Most of the discussion of the last two days has understandably surrounded circumstances in the United States. But I would underline the
fact that our problems really represent a microcosm of the health problems of the world at large. There are 200 million people in the world
who suffer from schistosomiasis. I submit that is a problem that, in
terms of any of us in this room, is more important than the problem of
cancer because the people who suffer from this condition, in general, are
much younger, have many more obligations to the people around them, and
for a variety of other reasons. Malaria is said to afflict almost a
million people. This is one facet of the problem that we do not look
at nearly so much in the United States as we might. Another is the
fact that the restraints that have been forced upon us to some extent,
that we have accepted in this country, have resulted in our going outside of the United States to evade them. That, too, is a responsibility
for us to examine in some detail, and to ask how or whether we should
tolerate it.

I think anybody who has been here for these two days has been struck
by the fact that by and large there have been two groups of people who
have been speaking. One group is the medical researchers, who feel
that the excesses, while they exist, are in general minimal as compared
with the dividends that have been brought to all of us. I accept that
point. They also feel that if the ground rules are changed appreciably,
research itself may be threatened. They feel, finally, that the other
players on the stage, potential or real, lawyers, chemists, social
workers, consumers, have no greater expertise, and often lesser expertise, than physicians or the investigators; and therefore, why change?

The second group is the nonphysicians, who are, in general, cogni-
zant of the contributions of medical research, but who are concerned
about the abrogation of individual rights.

We will get relatively little out of the events of the last two days
unless we recognize that this gulf is not going to be bridged unless we
find mechanisms for establishing a continuing dialogue between all of
the people who are concerned, a dialogue that introduces each of the
people involved to the problems, the aspirations, and the concerns of
the others. I am convinced that this can be done.

Over the last two years in Boston, we have succeeded in bringing
together a group of people, many of whom are members of this Forum,
for this purpose. At the outset of this continuing dialogue we had as
great difficulties in understanding each other as we have had here in
the last two days. And yet from this has emerged working groups involving people from law, medicine, philosophy, management, consumer
areas, and others as well, that have resulted in joint research efforts,
in joint approaches to old problems, in suggestions concerning new
problems. This seems to me to be very promising.

If, as a result of this session, the Academy and the Institute of
Medicine, or some other mechanism, can decide or will decide that this

problem is as important or perhaps more important than any other that confronts society, and as a result determines that some kind of a continuing body will be put together with a mission to bring forward a code in a given period of time, and to keep that code updated as time evolves, then this will all have been useful.

In my view, one needs no crystal ball to predict that rules and regulations will be forthcoming. There is ample evidence. A society that was sufficiently aroused to put together a Food and Drug Administration some six decades ago is going to do something about the unregulated medical and surgical procedures, and the relatively little-regulated medical research that goes on.

If what emerges from these regulations is to retain the best of what we have at the present time and to reflect the input of the clinical investigators, it seems to me that it must be they who take the lead in demonstrating the need for openness in the most real sense that one can project this term, that is, in partnership, involving themselves and all other interested groups, and putting forward the suggestions that might lead to a serious dealing with the problems that have concerned us.

FREDERICK ROBBINS

First, I cannot say strongly enough that I do not believe that biomedical research is necessarily threatened because we are discussing the problem, talking about the possibility of certain regulations, and concerned about abuses that have occurred. I would regard that as a strength, not a weakness. I think that a defensive point of view on the part of investigators is improper and unnecessary. If we have not proved our worth, then perhaps we should not proceed.

Secondly, our greatest obligation is to do good science, and many of the abuses have not been good science. As I said earlier, I am not convinced that some of what are considered abuses are true ones. On the other hand, I know there are abuses. And the fact that Dr. Chalkley is able to point to no legal actions and so on does not mean there are no abuses.

The kind of scrutiny that is going on now, by means of our various review committees, is perfectly in concert with the scientific method. I know, and you know, that the reason the scientific method was developed was because an investigator cannot trust himself always to interpret the results of an experiment in which he has invested a good bit of his ideas and his hypotheses. That is why you set up controls in experiments. The same principle applies in asking that others review your protocol before you embark on an experiment that involves other people. That seems like no great threat to me.

We have been using institutional review committees now for some time. I was impressed with Mr. Halpern's suggestion that we need to take a more investigative approach to what we have achieved, how are we doing, et cetera, the kind of thing that Ivan Bennett commented upon to some extent.

The need for a surrogate for children and other people who cannot give permission is clear and necessary, unless we say no investigation upon children or anybody else who cannot give consent themselves. I am not sure from what I heard, and from what I know is going on in this country, that we really want to do that, but we do need a surrogate.

I firmly believe that the kind of interchange now going on in the institutions, through the medium of the review committees, which are expanding themselves and experimenting to some extent but not enough, is beginning to develop the kind of relationship that Dr. Hiatt spoke about. Furthermore, it is beginning to have some impact in the educational system, and I feel very strongly that here is a most important area where we have to make every effort to be certain that those people whom we are educating, not just doctors, but people who are going to be involved in the investigation, understand the issues and are helped to see the problems through other people's eyes.

In closing I would like to quote from Hans Jonas and his article on "Philosophical Reflections on Human Experimentation" in the Spring 1969 issue of *Daedalus*. He has this to say about research:

> The destination of research is essentially melioristic. It does not serve the preservation of the existing good from which I profit myself and to which I am obligated. Unless the present state is intolerable, the melioristic goal is in a sense gratuitous, and not only from the vantage point of the present. Our descendents have a right to be left an unplundered planet; they do not have a right to new miracle cures.

Jonas then goes on to make this comment, one that we might keep in mind as we continue the deliberations of this Forum in our daily lives and work:

> . . . progress, with all our methodical labor for it, cannot be budgeted in advance and its fruits received as a due. Its coming about at all and its turning out for good (of which we can never be sure) must rather be regarded as something akin to grace.

That, I think, is an appropriate benediction for our experience here together over these past two day.

LEWIS THOMAS

I have been sitting here as the Chairman -- what Gilbert and Sullivan referred to as a tremendous swell in one context -- and we have run out

222

of time. Moreover, all of the sage spontaneous and extemporary remarks
that I so carefully prepared have already been made by my colleagues,
and I find myself in agreement with all of them, including, I must say,
Dr. Hiatt, and we are at peace.

I would like to extend thanks on behalf of everyone involved in this
Forum to this valiant and resilient audience for the devoted service
you have all put in. And now I would like to ask Dr. Handler if he will
say to us a few concluding remarks.

CLOSING

Philip Handler

I would like to thank Dr. Thomas, Dr. Robbins, and all of you for being with us for these two days. I am not sure whether the issues were really joined. That still seems to be the most difficult problem for us in the design of a forum. If the issue is sufficiently polarized, those at the two poles find grave difficulty in actually confronting each other and speaking in terms they both recognize and out of value systems that they can share.

On the first day, there were moments when it seemed to me that some of you wished to discuss those issues that you deem profound, while others wished to discuss those issues they deem important, regardless of their profundity. From time to time, we came closer to joining the controversy, if controversy there really be.

I see no reason for those who have been in the forefront of medical research in our time to be defensive of either their accomplishments or their behavior. Nor, however, should they attempt to "put down" those who have joined in the swelling sense of emotion in the United States that has so changed our world in the last ten years -- the sense of individual rights, of civil rights, the rights of those special groups in our population whom we have ignored too long, the sense of responsibility for the land in which we dwell, and even the growing sense of responsibility for those in other lands.

This morning when he opened the meeting, Dr. Fredrickson was voicing the question I posed when this meeting was planned. I asked, "How is it that when the death rate due to starvation is running about 12,000 a week in the rest of the world, you can sit here and worry about whether or not an unwanted fetus is or is not 'a person' at some specific day in its life?"

223

I think you have all answered that question for yourselves. The fact that much of the world is ugly, the fact that there are brutalizing forces, and always have been, should not deter us from seeking to determine that which is human and desirable, nor from asking what sort of world we would prefer to have, if we could but know it.

That, I think, is what you have been doing for these two days. Those of you who were on the two sides of this rather polarized meeting did, I think, find a little sense of what the others are about. If that facilitates a dialogue in the years ahead, this Forum was successful since that was all we were attempting to do.

NOTES AND REFERENCES

FRANCIS D. MOORE

1. Boylston, Z. An historical account of the smallpox inoculated in
    New England. London, 1726.
2. Paul, J. R. *A History of Poliomyelitis*. Yale University Press,
    New Haven and London, 1971.
3. Curran, W. J. Experimentation becomes a crime: Fetal research in
    Massachusetts. *New Engl. J. Med.* 292:300-301, 1975.
4. Katz, S. I., *et al.* Attenuated measles vaccine in Nigerian
    children. *Am. J. Dis. Child.* 103:402-406, 1952.
5. Moore, F. D. Transplant. *The Give and Take of Tissue Trans-
    plantation*. Simon and Schuster, New York, 1972.
6. Morain, W. D. Krebiozen: Nineteen years of controversy. Unpub-
    lished essay, Boylston Medical Society, Harvard Medical School
    (March 18, 1968).
7. Moore, F. D. Therapeutic innovation: Ethical boundaries in the
    initial clinical trials of new drugs and surgical procedures.
    Daedalus:502-522, 1969.
8. *Choroba Glodowa*. Published by the American Joint Distribution
    Committee, Warsaw, 1946. Apfelbaum, E., ed.

RENÉE C. FOX

1. Fox, Renée C. Ethical and existential developments in contemporan-
    eous American medicine: Their implications for culture and society.
    Milbank Memorial Foundation Quarterly, *Health and Society* (Fall
    1974):445-483.

225

2. Kass, Leon R. Making babies -- The new biology and the "old" morality. *The Public Interest* 26(Winter):32.

LEON EISENBERG

1. Freedman, A. M. Personal Communication.
2. Corner, G. W. (ed.) *The Autobiography of Benjamin Rush.* Princeton, Princeton University Press, 1948. Middleton, W.S. The yellow fever epidemic of 1793 in Philadelphia. *Ann. Med. Hist.* 10:434-450, 1928. Rush, B. *Medical Inquiries and Observations.* Philadelphia, 1809 (reprinted by Hafner, N.Y., 1962).
3. Eisenberg, L. The ethics of intervention: Acting amidst ambiguity. *J. Child Psychol. Psychiat.* In press, 1975.
4. Smith, W. C. Hypothetical protocol. This Forum, 1975.
5. Eisenberg, L. Principles of drug therapy in child psychiatry: With special reference to stimulant drugs. *Am. J. Orthopsychiat.* 41: 371-379, 1971.
6. Herbst, A. L., Uhlfelder, H., and Poskanzer, D. C. A denocarcinoma of the vagina: Association of maternal stilbesterol therapy with tumor appearance in young women. *N. Engl. J. Med.* 284:878-881, 1971. Herbst, A. L., *et al.* Clear-cell adenocarcinoma of the vagina and cervix in girls. *Am. J. Obstet. Gynecol.* 119:713-724, 1974. Herbst, A. L., *et al.* Prenatal exposure to stilbesterol: A prospective comparison of exposed female offspring with unexposed controls. *N. Engl. J. Med.* 292:334-339, 1975.
7. Harris, G. W. Sex hormones, brain development and brain function. *Endocrin.* 75:627-648, 1964. Jost, A. Sex differentiation in mammals. *Johns Hopkins Med. J.* 130:38-53, 1972. Karsch, F. J., *et al.* Sexual differentiation of pituitary function. *Science* 179:484, 1973. Raisman, G., and Field, P. M. Sexual dimorphism in the preoptic area of the rat. *Science* 173:731-733, 1973.
8. Michaels, R. P. (ed.) *Endocrinology and Human Behavior.* London, Oxford University Press, 1968. Money, J., and Erhardt, A. A. *Man and Woman, Boy and Girl.* Baltimore, Johns Hopkins Press, 1972. Luttge, W. G. The role of gonadal hormones in the sexual behavior of the Rhesus monkey. *Arch. Sex. Behav.* 1:61-88, 1971.
9. Smith, W. C. Remarks. This Forum, 1975.

ALBERT B. SABIN

1. Morris, N., and Mills, M. Prisoners as laboratory subjects. *The Wall Street Journal,* April 2, 1974. "For example, last April, 96 of the 175 inmates of the Lancaster County, Pa. prison wrote to the local newspaper protesting the state's decision to stop all medical experiments on state prisoners. . . With these minimum safeguards [they listed three requirements] as a precondition to the ethical participation of this vulnerable group, we believe that medical

research in prisons can be beneficial to society, to the prison system, and not least to the prisoner himself."

2. Neva, F. A. Research with *Plasmodium falciparum* in volunteers (Reply). *J. Infect. Dis.* 130:314-315, 1974.
3. Wells, S. H., Kennedy, P., Kenny, J., Reznikoff, M., and Sheard, M. H. Pharmacological testing in a correctional institution, 1974. Charles C. Thomas, Publisher, Springfield, Illinois.
4. Lack, H. L. $20-a-day guinea pigs with a nose for medical research. *Baltimore Sun (Magazine Section)*, pp. 10-18, December 15, 1974.

ALVIN J. BRONSTEIN

1. The original statement by Mr. Bronstein contained references to specific individuals and institutions which have been deleted by the Academy. The following references to situations involving specific institutions and individuals were cited by Mr. Bronstein in his prepared remarks: Morris and Mills, Prisoners as Laboratory Subjects, *The Wall Street Journal*, April 2, 1974; Jay Katz, *Experimentation with Human Beings*, Russell Sage Foundation (1972), p. 13.
2. See generally: Jessica Mitford. *Kind and Unusual Punishment* (Knopf, 1973); Ben H. Bagidikian. *The Shame of the Prisons* (Simon & Schuster, 1972); Erving Goffman. *Asylums* (Aldine, 1961).
3. Brief for the United States as *Amicus Curiae*, p. 15, *Preiser v. Newkirk*, O.T. 1974, No. 74-107.
4. Report to the Secretary, Public Safety and Correctional Services, State of Maryland, from the Governing Board of Patuxent Institution, p. 14, January 31, 1975.
5. See generally: David Rothman. Decarcerating prisoners and patients. *The Civial Liberties Review*, Fall 1973; Robert Martinson. What works? - Questions and answers about prison reform. *The Public Interest*, No. 35, Spring 1974 (To be published in early 1975 by Praeger in an expanded version as *The Effectiveness of Correctional Treatment*.); Edward M. Opton, Jr. *Psychiatric Violence Against Prisoners: When Therapy is Punishment*, 45 Miss. L. J. 605, 1974.
6. For example, State Prison of Southern Michigan at Jackson; Stateville Correctional Center at Joliet, Illinois.
7. Resource Document #4, Parole Corrections Project (American Correctional Association, March 1974), Table IV.
8. Id.
9. See generally: Alvin J. Bronstein. Rules for playing God. *The Civil Liberties Review*, Summer 1974.
10. Brief for the United States as *Amicus Curiae*, supra note 5, p. 30.
11. Quoted in Morris and Mills, *supra*, note 1.
12. Opton, *supra*, note 7.
13. Id.
14. *Knecht v. Gillman*, 488 F.2d 1136 (8th Cir. 1973).
15. *Clonce v. Richardson*, 379 F. Supp. 338 (W. D. Mo. 1974).

228

WILLIAM N. HUBBARD, JR.

1. Proceedings of the Conference on Drug Research in Prisons.
    National Council on Crime and Delinquency, August 1973.
2. Wells, S. H., Kennedy, P. M., *et al. Pharmacological Testing in a
    Correctional Institution.* Charles C. Thomas, 1974.
3. Clinical Pharmacology and the Human Volunteer, L. Lasagna, Chairman,
    Clin. Pharm. and Therap. Vol. 13, No. 5, Part 2, 1972.

GENERAL ADVISORY COMMITTEE

Robert McC. Adams, Dean, Division of Social Sciences, The University of Chicago, *Chairman*
Daniel E. Koshland, Jr., Professor & Chairman, Department of Biochemistry, University of California, Berkely, *Acting Chairman*
Arthur M. Bueche, Vice President, Corporate Research and Development, General Electric Company
Norman H. Giles, Callaway Professor of Genetics, Department of Zoology, University of Georgia
Gertrude S. Goldhaber, Senior Physicist, Brookhaven National Laboratory
Michael Kasha, Director, Institute of Molecular Biophysics, Florida State University
Rudolf Kompfner, Professor, Department of Engineering Science, University of Oxford, England
Philip Morrison, Institute Professor, Department of Physics, Massachusetts Institute of Technology
Frederick C. Robbins, Dean, School of Medicine, Case Western Reserve University
Lewis Thomas, President, Memorial Sloan-Kettering Cancer Center
Donald S. Fredrickson, President, Institute of Medicine, *Ex-Officio*
Robert C. Seamans, Jr., President, National Academy of Engineering, *Ex-Officio*

FORUM STAFF

Robert R. White, Director
M. Virginia Davis, Administrative Assistant
Betsy S. Turvene, Editor

229

Frederick C. Robbins, Dean, School of Medicine, Case Western Reserve
University, Cochairman
Lewis Thomas, President, Memorial Sloan-Kettering Cancer Center,
Cochairman
Lawrence K. Altman, Medical Writer, *New York Times*
Robert Austrian, John Herr Musser Professor & Chairman, Department of
Research Medicine, University of Pennsylvania
Richard E. Behrman, Carpentier Professor & Chairman, Department of
Pediatrics, College of Physicians and Surgeons, Columbia University
William J. Curran, Professor, Harvard School of Public Health
Renée C. Fox, Professor & Chairman, Department of Sociology, Univer-
sity of Pennsylvania
Samuel Gorovitz, Professor & Chairman, Department of Philosophy,
University of Maryland
Andre 'E. Hellegers, Director, Joseph and Rose Kennedy Institute for
the Study of Human Reproduction and Bioethics
Howard H. Hiatt, Dean, Harvard School of Public Health
William N. Hubbard, Jr., President, The Upjohn Company
Peter B. Hutt, Assistant Counsel, Food and Drug Division, Department
of Health, Education, and Welfare
William C. Smith, Staff Attorney, Children's Defense Fund
Sumner J. Yaffe, Professor of Pediatrics, Children's Hospital, Buffalo,
and Chairman, Committee on Drugs of the American Academy of Pediatrics

PARTICIPANTS

_____

SPEAKERS

Charles A. Alford, Jr., Meyer Professor of Pediatric Research, Department of Pediatrics and Microbiology, University of Alabama

Frederick C. Battaglia, Professor & Chairman, Department of Pediatrics, University of Colorado Medical Center

Richard E. Behrman, Carpentier Professor & Chairman, Department of Pediatrics, College of Physicians and Surgeons, Columbia University

Ivan L. Bennett, Jr., Provost, New York University Medical Center & Dean, New York University School of Medicine

Douglas D. Bond, Professor of Psychiatry, Case Western Reserve University

Alvin J. Bronstein, Executive Director-Counsel, National Prison Project, American Civil Liberties Union Foundation

Audrey K. Brown, Professor of Pediatrics & Physician-in-Charge, Pediatric Hematology-Oncology, Downstate Medical Center, State University of New York, Brooklyn

Leon Eisenberg, Professor of Psychiatry, Harvard Medical School & Senior Associate in Psychiatry, Children's Hospital Medical Center

Henry W. Foster, Professor & Chairman, Department of Obstetrics and Gynecology, George W. Hubbard Hospital, Meharry Medical College

Renée C. Fox, Professor & Chairman, Department of Sociology, University of Pennsylvania

Donald S. Fredrickson, President, Institute of Medicine

Charles Fried, Professor of Law, Harvard University Law School

Charles R. Halpern, Executive Director, Council for the Advancement of Public Interest Law

Philip Handler, President, National Academy of Sciences

231

232

Howard H. Hiatt, Dean, Harvard School of Public Health
Maurice R. Hilleman, Vice President, Merck Sharp & Dohme Research
  Laboratories
William N. Hubbard, Jr., President, The Upjohn Company
Franz J. Ingelfinger, Editor, New England Journal of Medicine
Robert B. Jaffe, Professor & Chairman, Department of Obstetrics and
  Gynecology, University of California Medical School, San Francisco
Jay Katz, Professor (Adjunct) of Law and Psychiatry, Yale Law School
Charles U. Lowe, Executive Director, The National Commission for the
  Protection of Human Subjects of Biomedical and Behavioral Research
Walsh McDermott, Special Advisor to the President of The Robert Wood
  Johnson Foundation
Richard A. Merrill, Associate Dean & Professor of Law, University of
  Virginia School of Law
Francis D. Moore, Moseley Professor of Surgery, Harvard Medical School
  & Surgeon-in-Chief, Peter Bent Brigham Hospital
Frederick C. Robbins, Dean, School of Medicine, Case Western Reserve
  University, Cochairman
Albert B. Sabin, Distinguished Research Professor of Biomedicine,
  Medical University of South Carolina
William C. Smith, Staff Attorney, Children's Defense Fund
Lewis Thomas, President, Memorial Sloan-Kettering Cancer Center,
  Cochairman
Caspar W. Weinberger, Secretary, Department of Health, Education, and
  Welfare

DISCUSSANTS

Lawrence K. Altman, Medical Writer, New York Times
Robert Austrian, John Herr Musser Professor & Chairman, Department of
  Research Medicine, University of Pennsylvania
Bernard Barber, Professor and Chairman, Department of Sociology,
  Barnard College, Columbia University
David L. Bazelon, Chief Judge of the United States Court of Appeals for
  the District of Columbia Circuit
Henry K. Beecher, Dorr Professor of Research in Anaesthesia, Emeritus,
  Harvard Medical School
Joseph Bellanti, Professor of Pediatrics & Microbiology, Georgetown
  University Hospital
Edward L. Buescher, Col. MC, Director, Walter Reed Army Institute of
  Research
Robert A. Burt, Professor, University of Michigan Law School
Alexander M. Capron, Assistant Professor of Law, University of Pennsyl-
  vania Law School
Frederick S. Carney, Professor of Ethics, Graduate Program in Religion,
  Southern Methodist University
D. T. Chalkley, Chief, Office for Protection from Research Risks,
  Office of the Director, National Institutes of Health

James F. Childress, Chairman, Department of Religious Studies, University of Virginia
William J. Curran, Professor, Harvard School of Public Health
William J. Darby, President, The Nutrition Foundation
Albert Dorfman, Richard T. Crane Distinguished Service Professor of Pediatrics and Biochemistry, University of Chicago
Arthur J. Dyck, Mary B. Saltonstall Professor of Population Ethics, Harvard School of Public Health
Erwin A. France, Administrative Assistant to the Mayor of Chicago
H. Hugh Fudenberg, Professor and Chairman, Department of Basic and Clinical Immunology and Microbiology, Medical University of South Carolina; Professor of Medicine, University of California School of Medicine, San Francisco; and Professor of Immunology, University of California, Berkeley
Willard Gaylin, President, Institute of Society, Ethics and the Life Sciences
Joan Goldstein, Task Force on Women and Health, National Organization for Women
Samuel Gorovitz, Professor & Chairman, Department of Philosophy, University of Maryland
Robert E. Greenberg, Professor and Chairman, Department of Pediatrics, Charles R. Drew Postgraduate Medical School, and President, Society for Pediatric Research
Michael J. Halberstam, Associate Clinical Professor of Internal Medicine and Cardiology, George Washington University Hospital
Elizabeth D. Hay, Louise Foote Pfeiffer Professor of Embryology, Department of Anatomy, Harvard Medical School
Andre 'E. Hellegers, Director, Joseph and Rose Kennedy Institute for the Study of Human Reproduction and Bioethics
John H. Knowles, President, The Rockefeller Foundation
Saul Krugman, Professor, Department of Pediatrics, New York University Medical Center
Irving Ladimer, Special Counsel in Health Care, American Arbitration Association
Louis C. Lasagna, Professor and Chairman, Department of Pharmacology and Toxicology, University of Rochester School of Medicine and Dentistry
Brian Little, Professor and Chairman, Department of Reproductive Biology, Case Western Reserve University School of Medicine
Richard A. McCormick, S.J., Rose F. Kennedy Professor of Christian Ethics, Joseph and Rose Kennedy Institute for the Study of Human Reproduction and Bioethics
Gerard Piel, Publisher, *The Scientific American*
Barbara Rosenkrantz, Associate Professor, Department of the History of Science, Harvard University
Lois J. Schiffer, Attorney, Women's Rights Project, Center for Law and Social Policy
George E. Schreiner, Professor of Medicine, Georgetown University Hospital

234

DeWitt Stetten, Jr., Deputy Director for Science, National Institutes
of Health
Christine Stevens, President, Animal Welfare Institute
John W. Tukey, Bell Laboratories
Marie A. Valdes-Dapena, Associate Pathologist, St. Christopher's
Hospital for Children; Professor of Pathology and Professor in
Pediatrics, Temple University School of Medicine
Sheldon M. Wolff, Clinical Director, National Institute of Allergy and
Infectious Diseases
Theodore Woodward, Professor and Chairman, Department of Medicine,
University of Maryland Hospital

This Academy Forum received support from:

The National Academy of Sciences
The Department of Health, Education, and Welfare
The National Endowment for the Humanities
The National Science Foundation

Abbott Laboratories
American Sheet Metal Workers' International Association
Baxter Laboratories, Inc.
Hoffmann-La Roche, Inc.
Johnson & Johnson
Lilly Research Laboratories, Division of Eli Lilly & Co.
Merck Sharp & Dohme Research Laboratories
Pfizer, Inc.
Schering-Plough Corporation
G. D. Searle & Co.
Smith Kline & French Laboratories
Squibb Corporation
Sterling Drug, Inc.
The Upjohn Company